POWER
BOWLS

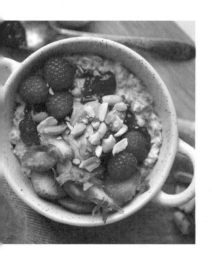
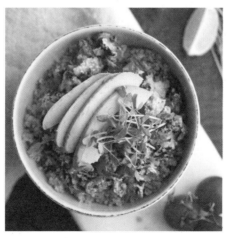
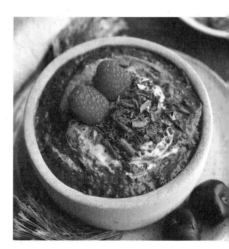

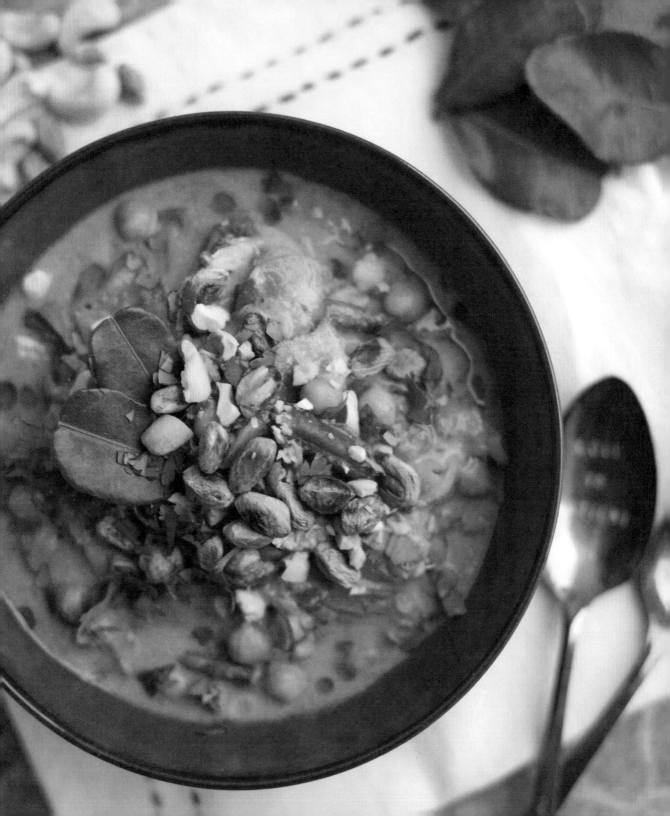

POWER BOWLS

100 PERFECTLY BALANCED MEALS IN A BOWL

CHRISTAL SCZEBEL, CHN

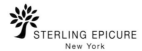

STERLING EPICURE
New York

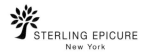

STERLING EPICURE
New York

An Imprint of Sterling Publishing Co., Inc.
1166 Avenue of the Americas
New York, NY 10036

ISBN 978-1-4549-2699-3

Distributed in Canada by Sterling Publishing Co., Inc.
c/o Canadian Manda Group, 664 Annette Street
Toronto, Ontario, Canada M6S 2C8
Distributed in the United Kingdom by GMC Distribution Services
Castle Place, 166 High Street, Lewes, East Sussex, England BN7 1XU
Distributed in Australia by NewSouth Books
45 Beach Street, Coogee, NSW 2034, Australia

For information about custom editions, special sales, and premium and corporate purchases,
please contact Sterling Special Sales at 800-805-5489 or specialsales@sterlingpublishing.com.

Manufactured in China

2 4 6 8 10 9 7 5 3 1

sterlingpublishing.com

Written and photographed by Christal Sczebel

Contents

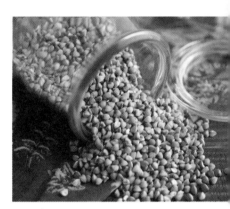

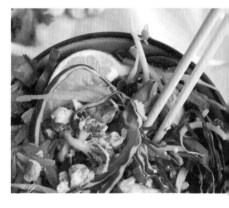

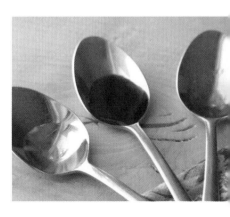

Introduction

When I began to write this book, I wasn't sure if many people would understand the term "power bowl," but I've been pleasantly surprised by the response. Now that we live in the Pinterest age, so many amazing recipes are at the tips of our fingers, and in the past couple of years power bowls have gained serious popularity. But what is it about power bowls—or "bowl food"—that makes it so great? A lot!

First of all, the options for bowl food are vast. A bowl is a magnificent dish because it can cradle everything from cold smoothies and savory soups to stewed goodies, fresh salads, and warm breakfasts. This means that the opportunity to fill a bowl with powerful, nutritionally dense, health-boosting, and vibrant ingredients is endless.

Secondly, bowl foods are simple. You can hold an array of health-promoting ingredients in your hand and enjoy them without the need for several dishes, or even a table and chair to eat at.

All the power bowls in this book follow a set of principles that makes them potent for the health of both body and mind. When I create a power bowl it always fits the following criteria:

• It contains mostly, if not all, whole food, unprocessed, natural ingredients.

• It contains an array of nutrients—vitamins, minerals, fiber, fats, carbohydrates, and proteins.

• It combines different textures and tastes (there are no one-dimensional dishes here!).

• It contains all three macronutrients—proteins, carbohydrates, and fats.

• It doesn't take rocket science to put together.

• It tastes amazing!

I also like to make my power bowls allergen-friendly, meaning that most of the recipes are free from the two main food allergens: dairy and gluten. If they aren't, you can easily make a substitution. (See Ingredient Substitutions on page 184.)

In each chapter you'll find a power bowl to fit into your day. There are Wake Up Bowls to start you off on the right foot; Workout Bowls to be enjoyed before or after exercise to fuel your body or help it recover from the activity; Small Bowls to supply a nutritional punch for a light lunch or larger snack later in the day; Big Bowls, for larger appetites, to provide major fuel any time of day; and, finally, Treat Bowls to satisfy your sweet tooth, while still providing an ample amount of nutrients for optimal wellness.

CHRISTAL SCZEBEL

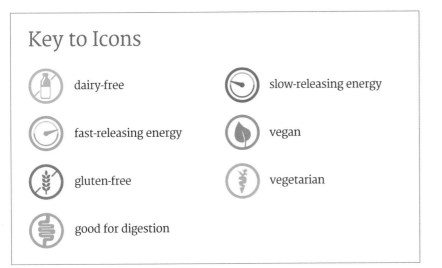

Key to Icons

- dairy-free
- fast-releasing energy
- gluten-free
- good for digestion
- slow-releasing energy
- vegan
- vegetarian

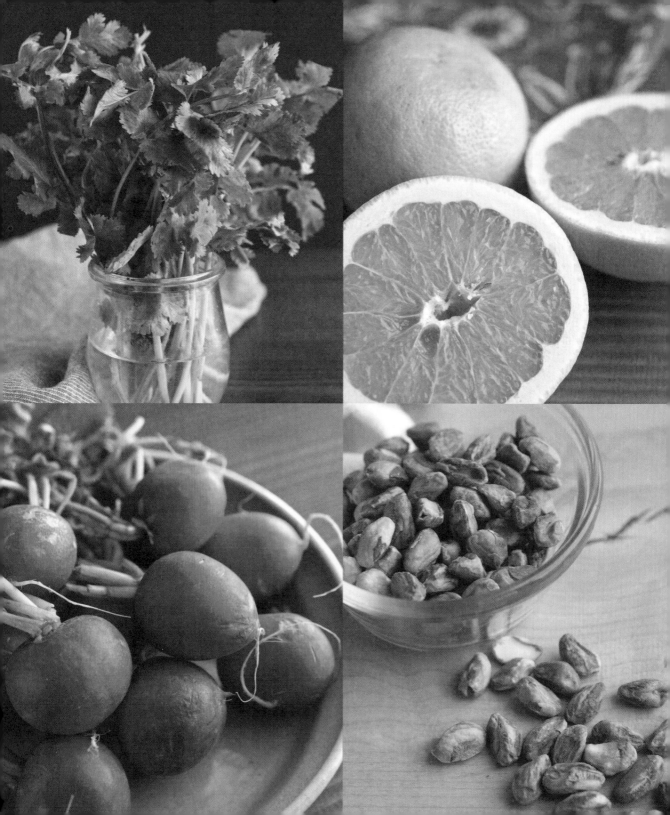

PART ONE

Power Bowl Basics

Good nutrition is important, if you want your body to be healthy. To do this, you need to use the best ingredients and know how to prepare them. If you are following a special diet, there are a number of things you need to take into account when preparing meals.

Eating to Power Your Body

It's important to think of your body as an amazing and complex machine that needs to be fueled adequately and cared for throughout the day. Nutrition plays a huge part in this. For example, If you had a prized, powerful, and beautiful sports car you would prioritize putting premium products into it, especially the fuel. You should think of your body in the same way, and eating to power it should be of the utmost importance. Although you can enjoy indulgent foods on occasion, you should eat healthy, whole foods most of the time to keep your engine running smoothly.

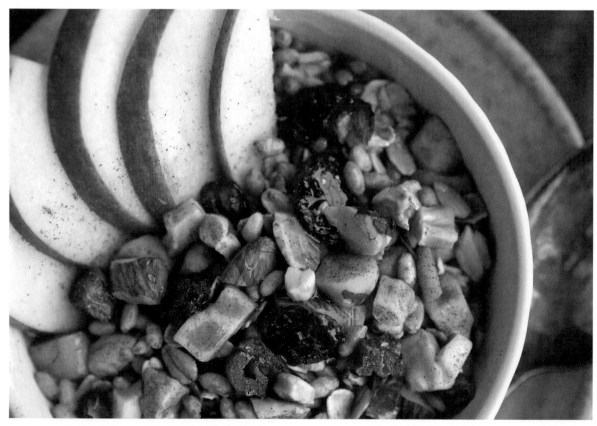

Start the day with a bowl of Apple Cinnamon (see page 69).

Breakfast

Eating to power your body starts as soon as you wake up. First, drink a glass of water for quick hydration. Filling your belly with healthy, hearty, and vibrant foods within one hour of waking will rev up your metabolism for fat-burning throughout the day, wake up your digestion, and provide the energy you need to get going and keep going. Starting the day with a focus on complex carbohydrates helps to fuel your body immediately and throughout the morning. These carbohydrates break down into sugars that act as direct fuel for energy. At the same time, if you incorporate protein and healthy fats into your breakfast, it will help balance blood sugars to keep that energy steady, as well as give you a sense of fullness and satiety.

Lunch

By midday your body is usually ready for another pick-me-up and a dose of well-balanced nutrition. Combining complex carbohydrates and loads of vegetables with proteins and some healthy fats will help keep your engine humming along. Include a balance of all three macronutrients (carbohydrates, protein, and fats) at this meal. Try to limit dietary fats, as eating excessive fat at lunch can make you feel sluggish and bogged down, creating afternoon sleepiness. However, fats are not "bad," and are essential to the body, so it is best to enjoy a moderate amount of healthy, unsaturated fats at lunchtime.

Dinner

When you are winding down in the evening, your body is usually ready for some extra TLC, and it's an ideal time to nourish it with vitamin- and mineral-rich vegetables, supportive and repairing proteins, healthy fats, and a moderate amount of complex carbohydrates to keep your energy steady throughout the evening. At dinner it's not uncommon for people to eat a heavy meal that overloads their digestion. Replacing this with a power bowl that's high in fiber, vegetables, lean proteins, and easily digested complex carbohydrates, will take the burden off and prevent you from feeling that you could plop on the couch and hit the hay for good.

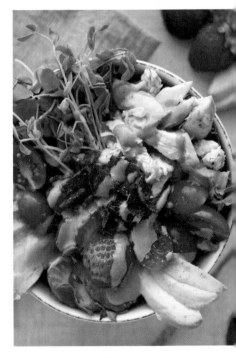

Proteins and vegetables are essential at lunchtime. Try a California Chicken & Avocado bowl (see page 120).

Between Meals

Your body will benefit from some added fuel through healthy snacks. These quick pick-me-ups help to stabilize blood sugar, maintain energy levels, keep cravings at bay, and power your metabolism between mealtimes. Protein is a key nutrient, paired with either healthy fats or carbohydrates. Workout bowls, small bowls, and even treat bowls, can be great snack options between meals on especially busy days.

When eating to power your body, it is important to choose foods that are whole and unprocessed, and as close to their natural state as possible. Foods that have been overly processed or contain additives, such as artificial flavorings or colorings, preservatives, and refined sweeteners, rob your body of energy, because it takes a lot of work for your body to detoxify and digest these foods. Your body acts like a sorting mechanism; when you consume food, your body's systems work together to make sure the right nutrients go to the right places, ensuring that it functions at its best. However, when your body is overloaded with ingredients that need to be eliminated, because they have no beneficial function, your sorting mechanism can become sluggish and inefficient, which saps your energy, strength, and ultimately your health.

When buying foods to power your body, you should focus on those that include minimal ingredients, little or no additives, and are fresh. Fruits, vegetables, meats, poultry, and seafood fall into this category, along with complex carbohydrates, such as whole grains, legumes, nuts, and seeds. These complex carbohydrates can be bought dried, canned, or fresh; just be sure there isn't a lengthy ingredients list on the label. Most of the ingredients used in power bowls can be kept in the refrigerator or freezer and some are nonperishables, which can be stored in the pantry.

This book has recipes that may be suitable for different seasons of the year. For example, a power bowl that's loaded with berries might be best to enjoy in the summer months, when berries are ripe and in season, potatoes might be more appropriate for the winter months. You'll get the most benefit from eating foods when they are in season.

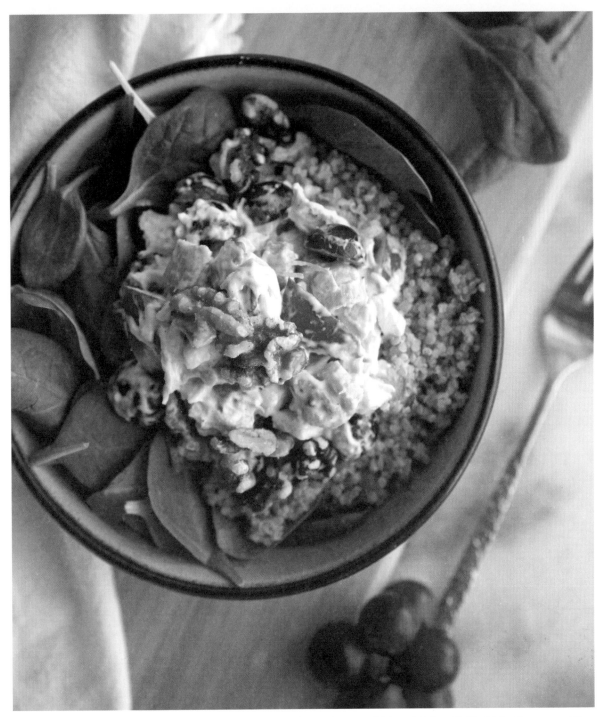

Leafy greens bring many nutritional benefits to a meal. Here, they enhance a Chicken & Quinoa Waldorf Salad (see page 126).

Ingredient Profiles:
Dairy

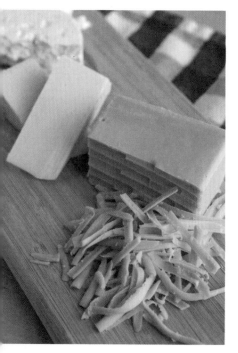

Selection of cheeses

Cheddar Cheese

Origin England
Food Family Dairy
Nutrients Calcium, magnesium, vitamins A, B12, D
Power Properties While I do not use Cheddar cheese often, it does add flavor, richness, and calcium to a dish. Look for organic brands that have no added artificial ingredients, flavors, coloring, or preservatives.

Cream Cheese and Alternatives

Origin First produced in the United States
Food Family Dairy/condiment
Nutrients Calcium, vitamins A, B12, D
Power Properties This softened cheese is typically made from a mixture of milk and cream, but you can find dairy-free varieties made from cashews, coconut oil, pea protein, and plant-based starches, such as tapioca or potato. Each type contains different nutrients. A small amount of this soft, decadent cheese adds creaminess, and its fats fill you up. When combined with fruit and natural sweeteners, the fat helps to slow down the release of carbohydrates and control your blood sugar. Buy plain cream cheeses with minimal ingredients that are recognizable and without added sugars or artificial ingredients.

Feta Cheese

Origin Greece
Food Family Dairy
Nutrients Calcium, fats, magnesium, protein, vitamins A, B6, B12, D
Power Properties Feta is a variety of white cheese traditionally made in Greece from sheep's milk, or a mixture of sheep and goat's milk. Varieties of feta cheese are also made with cow's milk in North America and areas of Europe. All feta cheeses are rich in minerals, including calcium and magnesium, as well as B vitamins and vitamin A.

Feta cheeses are also a source of dietary fats and proteins, making it a nutrient-filled dairy option. It adds a natural, salty flavor that complements vegetables, herbs, and proteins. Its best to choose an organic brand made with goat's or sheep's milk rather than cow's, as the likelihood of intolerance is much less and they tend to be digested more easily.

Mayonnaise

Origin Spain
Food Family Dairy/condiment
Nutrients Iron, omega fatty acids, vitamins A, B12, D
Power Properties This creamy dressing is traditionally made by emulsifying oil, egg yolk, vinegar or lemon juice, and seasonings. While there are many varieties, I use a simple, organic mayonnaise made with olive oil. This type is free from added sugars and preservatives, and contains omega-rich fatty acids. Mayonnaise adds healthy fats and great flavor to dressings. You can make your own mayonnaise, or look for a commercial organic brand with no added sugars, preservatives, coloring, or artificial ingredients.

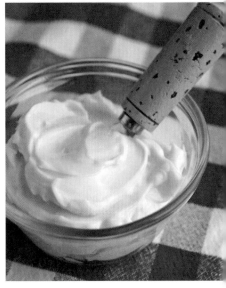
Mayonnaise

Sour Cream and Alternatives

Origin Eastern Europe, Germany, Ukraine, and Russia
Food Family Dairy
Nutrients Calcium, vitamins A, B6, B12, D
Power Properties Sour cream is traditionally made by fermenting regular cream with lactic acid bacteria in order to thicken it. Dairy-free sour creams are usually made from cashew, soy, or coconut milks, or from a mixture of plant-based oils and starches. Sour cream adds richness and creaminess to a dish. It has calcium, along with other minerals and vitamins. Try to use organic regular or dairy-free sour cream, with minimal, recognizable ingredients, and which does not contain any added sugars or artificial ingredients.

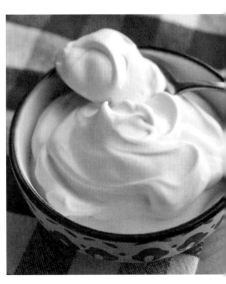
Sour cream

Ingredient Profiles:
Fats

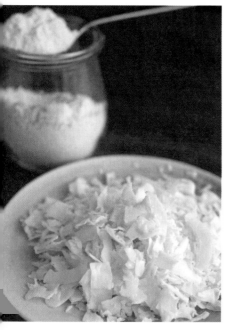

Coconut flour and flakes

Coconut Flour, Flakes, and Milk

Origin Southeast Asia

Food Family Palm tree

Nutrients Fiber, iron, magnesium, MCT (medium chain triglycerides) fats, vitamins B6, C

Power Properties Coconut is a versatile food and can be transformed into flour, shredded into flakes, or made into milk. All three forms make their way into the power bowls in this book, and each plays a different role. No matter how the coconut is used, it's a source of minerals, healthy fats, and fiber.

Coconut Oil

Origin Southeast Asia

Food Family Palm tree

Nutrients MCT (medium chain triglycerides) fats

Power Properties It's not surprising that coconut oil has received a lot of attention in the health world recently, as it has been linked to many health benefits. The medium chain triglycerides (MCTs) found in coconut oil have been shown to improve cardiovascular health, help combat diabetes, and improve weight management. Adding coconut oil to power bowls helps fill you up and adds dietary fats to a meal.

Olive Oil and Olives

Origin Unknown—thought to have been Northern Africa

Food Family Oleaceae

Nutrients Copper, unsaturated fats, fiber (in olives only), iron, vitamin E

Power Properties Olives, and the oil sourced from them, are loaded with unsaturated fats. The fats found in olives and olive oil have been linked to improved cardiovascular and nervous system health, reduced inflammation in the body, healthier hair, skin, and nails. Olives, which are naturally salty and fatty, add texture to power bowls. Olive oil is a wonderful choice for cooking proteins, roasting vegetables, and making dressings.

Sesame Oil

Origin Asia and Middle East

Food Family Pedaliaceae

Nutrients Unsaturated and saturated fats

Power Properties Derived from the mineral-rich sesame seed, this is a pungent oil that works well in Asian-inspired power bowls. It is naturally high in unsaturated fats and also contains some saturated fats to make you feel full. In small doses, sesame oil packs a punch of flavor and nutrition.

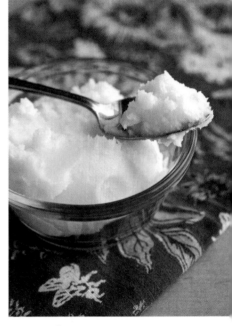

Coconut oil

Ingredient Profiles:
Meat, Poultry & Seafood

Bacon, Nitrate-Free

Origin Various
Food Family Animal
Nutrients Iron, magnesium, protein, vitamins B6, B12, D
Power Properties I bet you didn't think that bacon would make it onto a healthy food list, but if you're careful there's no reason why it shouldn't be included. Bacon is typically made from cured pork with added nitrates, which have been linked to cancer and other health problems. Luckily, bacon can be made without nitrates and from proteins other than pork, including beef and turkey. Try to find nitrate-free beef bacon that is locally sourced from grass-fed animals.

Breakfast Sausage

Origin First produced in the United States and Europe
Food Family Animal
Nutrients Iron, protein, vitamins B6, B12
Power Properties Breakfast sausage might not seem like the best power-giving food, but all sausages are not created equal. Nowadays, you can purchase organic and pasture-raised breakfast sausage made from leaner meats, such as chicken and turkey, and which are free of nitrates, artificial additives, and fillers. It is an awesome source of protein and helps maintain blood-sugar levels, fuel the body, and keep cravings at bay.

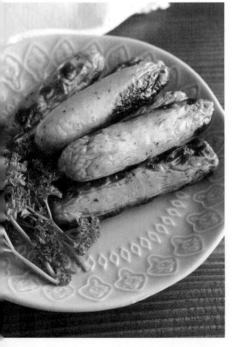

Breakfast Sausage

Chicken

Origin Southeast Asia
Food Family Fowl
Nutrients Magnesium, phosphorus, potassium, protein, selenium, vitamins B3, B5, B6, B12
Power Properties Chicken is an incredible source of protein, vitamins, and minerals. As well as fueling the body, protein from chicken helps to prevent fluctuations in blood-sugar levels, and

supports many of the body's systems. Different cuts contain varying amounts of saturated fat: the breast is the leanest cut, while chicken legs and thighs have more fat. All these cuts are beneficial, but it's recommended to use the chicken breast (with the skin removed), more often than the legs and thighs, and pair it with healthy unsaturated fats. Buy organic, humanely raised, free-range chicken, as it is the most nutrient-dense option.

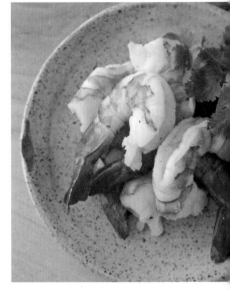

Shrimp

Shrimp

Origin Various
Food Family Crustacean
Nutrients Choline, copper, iodine, phosphorus, protein, selenium, vitamins B3, B12
Power Properties There are many health benefits to be gained from eating shrimp, including antioxidants that help the body defend against disease. These lean crustaceans are also an awesome source of protein that helps keep blood-sugar levels steady, prevent cravings, and support muscle growth and repair.

Turkey

Origin Americas
Food Family Phasianidae
Nutrients Iron, phosphorus, potassium, protein, zinc, vitamins B6, B12
Power Properties The protein found in turkey helps balance the carbohydrates and healthy fats in a dish, and also provides amino acids. It's also rich in minerals and B vitamins. Turkey breast meat is protein-dense and has fewer saturated fats than leg or thigh cuts. To balance blood sugar, improve energy, and support muscles, turkey is a great ingredient. Try to use organic, humanely raised, free-range turkey, as this is the best quality, most nutrient-dense option.

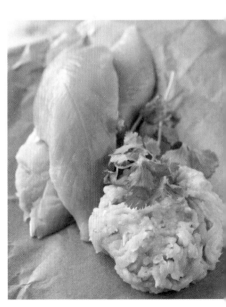

Turkey

Ingredient Profiles:
Complex Carbohydrates

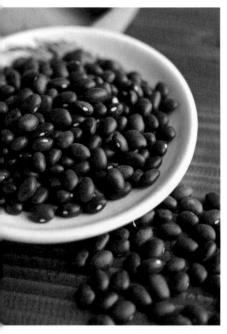

Black beans

Black Beans

Origin Americas
Food Family Legumes
Nutrients Carbohydrates, copper, folate, fiber, iron, manganese, magnesium, molybdenum, phosphorus, protein, vitamin B1
Power Properties Black beans are a superfood, thanks to their carbohydrates and fiber. They are also a source of plant-based protein, which contains many amino acids, minerals, and vitamins. You can buy black beans dried or canned. If you prefer canned beans, look for an organic brand that has no preservatives.

Bran, Spelt, Rice Flakes

Origin Various
Food Family Various
Nutrients Carbohydrates, fiber, iron, magnesium, manganese, B vitamins
Power Properties Many whole grains, including bran, rice, and spelt, are available as flakes, and are commonly used in breakfast cereals. Whole grains are an easy and tasty way to add slow-releasing complex carbohydrates to a dish and to give you sustained energy, fiber for fullness and digestion, and iron to strengthen and fortify your body. Choose whole-grain flakes without any added sugars or sweeteners.

Buckwheat Groats

Origin Central Asia

Food Family Polygonaceae

Nutrients Carbohydrates, copper, fiber, magnesium, manganese, phosphorus, B vitamins

Power Properties Buckwheat groats are a great ingredient, especially in wake up or workout bowls, they contain protein, including all of the essential amino acids, as well as slow-release, energizing, complex carbohydrates. They add a nice crunchy texture and nutty taste, too.

Chickpeas (Garbanzo Beans)

Origin Asia

Food Family Fabaceae

Nutrients Carbohydrates, copper, fiber, folate, iron, manganese, molybdenum, phosphorus, protein, zinc, vitamin B6

Power Properties These tasty legumes add protein and, as a complex carbohydrate, supply sustained energy. They also contain fiber, minerals, and vitamin B6. Chickpeas are a good option when you need quick energy. They are available in bulk, as dried beans, and require some prep, but, to save time, you can buy prepared, canned chickpeas.

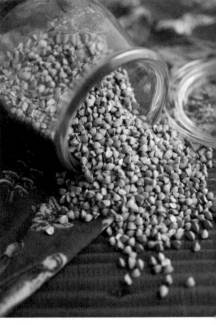

Buckwheat groats

Potatoes

Origin Multiple regions

Food Family Nightshade

Nutrients Carbohydrates, copper, fiber, manganese, potassium, vitamins B6, C

Power Properties Potatoes have a reputation for being a "bad carbohydrate," but that couldn't be farther from the truth. They provide carbohydrates for energy, fiber for digestion, as well as unique proteins, such as patatin, which protects against free radicals. The key is to eat them in a healthy way—not deep-fried! Roasted or sautéed potatoes provide energy and support digestion.

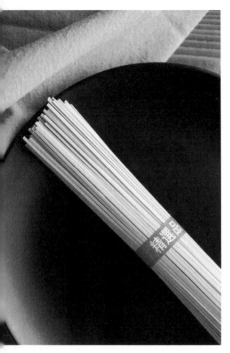

Soba noodles

Soba (Buckwheat) Noodles

Origin Central Asia

Food Family Polygonaceae

Nutrients Carbohydrates, copper, fiber, magnesium, manganese, phosphorus, B vitamins

Power Properties Soba noodles, also known as buckwheat noodles, are made from buckwheat flour. They are darker than egg or rice noodles and are often used in Asian-inspired dishes. They contain all the benefits of buckwheat, including mineral content, vitamins, fiber, and slow-releasing carbohydrates. When purchasing soba noodles, make sure they are made with 100 percent buckwheat flour and have no added refined flour.

Whole-grain & Gluten-free Pasta

Origin Various

Food Family Various

Nutrients Carbohydrates, iron, selenium, B vitamins, may also contain omega fatty acids

Power Properties Pasta has received a bad reputation over the years, but I don't believe that's warranted. When it is produced from simple whole grains (whether it's one grain or a mixture of them), pasta becomes a fantastic source of complex carbohydrates for slow-releasing, sustainable energy, filling you up and fueling your body for hours. Some whole-grain and gluten-free grain pastas even contain seeds like chia or flax that increase the omega-rich fat content. When choosing pasta, look for those that are made solely from whole grains, such as quinoa, rice, durum wheat, or amaranth. Avoid those with refined or "enriched" flours.

Ingredient Profiles:
Nuts & Seeds

Almonds, Almond Butter, Almond Milk, Almond Flour

Origin China and Central Asia

Food Family Rosaceae

Nutrients Biotin, copper, fats, fiber, phosphorus, magnesium, manganese, molybdenum, protein, vitamins B2, E

Power Properties Almonds, an incredibly versatile nut, are available in many forms, such as flour, butter, milk, and plain, raw nuts. Not only are they rich in vitamins and minerals, almonds are also a source of omega-rich fats and protein. They contain fiber and help keep hunger pangs at bay. Almonds are known to help support heart health, protect against disease, promote healthy weight management, and improve energy levels.

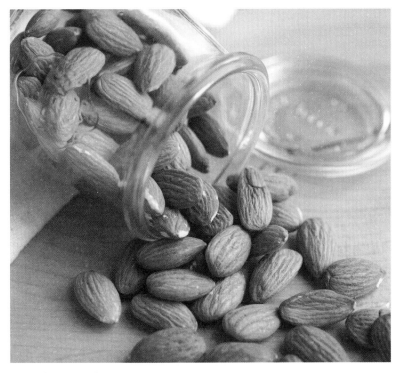

Almonds

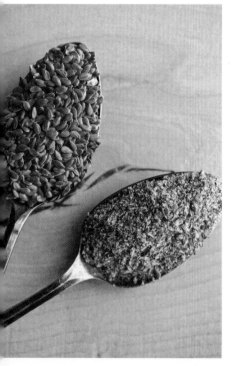

Flaxseed

Brazil Nuts

Origin South America

Food Family Bertholletia

Nutrients Calcium, fiber, iron, magnesium, protein, selenium, unsaturated fats

Power Properties These large, crunchy nuts, named after their country of origin, are full of minerals, and have awesome health benefits. One Brazil nut has the entire daily recommended dietary allowance of the mineral selenium, which helps thyroid health and has antioxidant and disease prevention benefits. Brazil nuts are also a source of unsaturated fats and help stabilize blood-sugar levels, as well as create a feeling of satiety.

Cashews

Origin Brazil

Food Family Anacardiaceae

Nutrients Copper, magnesium, manganese, monounsaturated fats, phosphorus, protein, zinc

Power Properties Cashews are rich in dietary fats, proteins, and minerals, including magnesium and zinc. They have been linked to heart health. The copper found in cashews also helps improve energy levels, support bones, and has an antioxidant effect. You can use cashews in sauces, as they create a wonderfully creamy consistency when blended, adding richness and flavor, as well as nutrients.

Flaxseed

Origin Believed to be Egypt

Food Family Linaceae

Nutrients Calcium, fiber, iron, magnesium, vitamin B6

Power Properties Historically, flaxseed was valued for it medicinal properties, as a laxative, an anti-inflammatory to control coughs, and even as a pain reliever. In a power bowl, its fiber content stimulates and supports digestion. Use ground flaxseed, which has the consistency of flour and is easier to digest than whole flaxseed, making it a better option for those who have sensitive digestive systems.

Hazelnuts

Origin Thought to be China
Food Family Corylus
Nutrients Calcium, fats, iron, magnesium, protein, vitamins B6,C, E
Power Properties Hazelnuts, also known as filberts, contain vitamins and minerals, along with healthy, filling fats. They are also a source of plant-based protein, with around 20g of protein per cup. Hazelnuts have been shown to control appetite, stabilize blood sugars, enhance energy, and help support the nervous system.

Hempseed

Origin Central Asia
Food Family Cannabis
Nutrients Fiber, iron, magnesium, omega fatty acids, potassium, protein, vitamin E
Power Properties Hempseeds are loaded with protein, which makes them a fantastic energizer. They also contain fiber, essential fatty acids, iron, magnesium, potassium, and antioxidants including vitamin E. While hempseeds are part of the cannabis family, eating them won't alter your mood, as they are different from the plant used to produce marijuana.

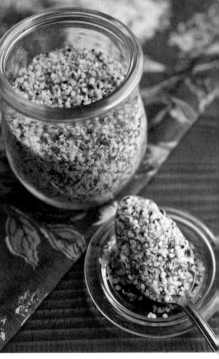

Hempseed

Peanuts and Peanut Butter

Origin South America
Food Family Legumes
Nutrients Copper, folate, manganese, molybdenum, monosaturated fats, protein, vitamin B3
Power Properties Although peanuts and peanut butter contain fat and calories, active people need these—along with protein—to prevent muscle density loss. Anyone who participates in endurance exercise will benefit from adding peanuts to their diet (as long as they do not have an intolerance or allergy to peanuts). When choosing peanuts, raw or dry-roasted are best. You can make your own peanut butter by grinding raw peanuts, or purchase a brand that has no added sugars, oils, or salt.

Pecans

Origin North America and Mexico
Food Family Juglandaceae
Nutrients Calcium, iron, magnesium, monosaturated fats, vitamin B6
Power Properties These rich, filling, buttery nuts are full of minerals and healthy, unsaturated fatty acids, including oleic acid, known to help promote healthy cholesterol levels. Pecans are also rich in antioxidants to help combat disease and inflammation in the body. They make a crunchy, filling, blood-sugar balancing, healthy ingredient. They are also wonderful when combined with chocolate, and can be enjoyed in sweet and savory dishes.

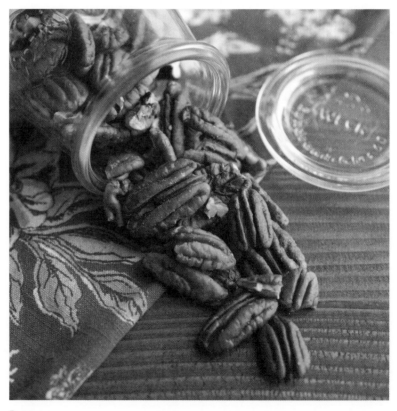

Pecans

Pistachios

Origin Asia
Food Family Anacardiaceae
Nutrients Copper, fats, iron, manganese, phosphorus, protein, vitamins B1, B6, E,
Power Properties These delicious nuts add a healthy crunch, energy-improving properties, skin and hair support, and antioxidant power to a dish. Their green hue comes from the lutein found in the nut, a carotenoid that has been shown to aid eye health. Use shelled, unsalted, or lightly salted pistachios.

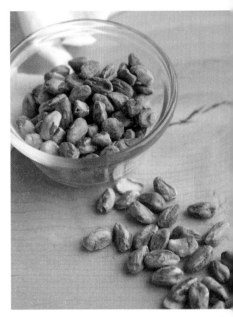

Pistachios

Sesame Seeds

Origin Asia and Middle East
Food Family Pedaliaceae
Nutrients Copper, fats, calcium, iron, magnesium, manganese, phosphorus, zinc
Power Properties When it comes to sources of plant-based calcium, sesame seeds are top-notch. Just 1/4 cup of these seeds contains 35 percent of the daily recommended dietary allowance of calcium. They help improve health in many ways, including strengthening bones, supporting the heart, and acting as an anti-inflammatory. Sesame seeds taste great, especially when lightly toasted.

Walnuts

Origin Persia and North America
Food Family Juglandaceae
Nutrients Biotin, copper, fats, manganese, molybdenum
Power Properties This oily nut is a nutrient powerhouse. Just 1/4 cup contains 113 percent of the daily recommended dietary allowance of omega-3 fatty acids, which are known to support nervous system and heart health. These healthy fats are filling and help keep blood-sugar levels stable, while increasing energy and stamina.

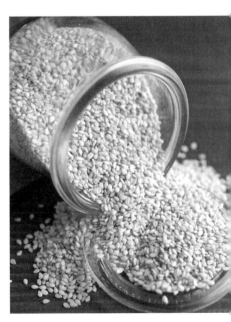

Sesame seeds

Ingredient Profiles:
Vegetables

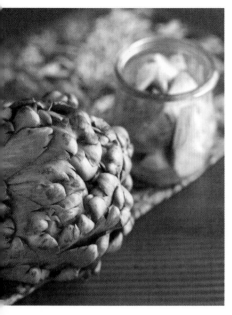

Artichokes

Artichokes

Origin Mediterranean
Food Family Daisy
Nutrients Fiber, folate, magnesium, manganese, potassium, vitamins C, K
Power Properties Artichokes are often skipped over in the vegetable section, but definitely shouldn't be. They are full of nutrients and antioxidants to help the immune system, prevent disease, and reduce inflammation. Artichokes are also a source of dietary fiber to keep you fueled and feeling full for hours. For convenience, use organic, canned artichoke hearts, with no added preservatives or artificial ingredients.

Arugula

Origin Mediterranean
Food Family Cabbage
Nutrients Calcium, folate, magnesium, manganese, vitamins A, C, K
Power Properties This spicy, sharp-tasting leafy green is loaded with vitamins, particularly vitamin K, minerals, and even provides some fiber and plant proteins. Also known as "garden rocket," arugula is known to enhance the body's detoxification process and has been linked to lower cholesterol and blood pressure, low inflammation, and improved blood flow. This heart-healthy green adds flavor and texture, too.

Bell Peppers

Origin Mexico, Central and South America
Food Family Nightshade
Nutrients Fiber, folate, molybdenum, vitamins A, B6, C, E
Power Properties Crunchy, colorful, sweet, and filling, bell peppers add bulk and loads of antioxidants, vitamins, and minerals to a meal. They are particularly high in carotenoids, which give them their bright hue, but more importantly, carotenoids are specific antioxidant

phytonutrients that are linked to disease and cancer prevention and improved immunity and health. Yellow, orange, red, and green bell peppers work well in power bowls.

Broccoli

Origin Mediterranean and Asia
Food Family Cabbage
Nutrients Chromium, fiber, folate, vitamins C and K
Power Properties Broccoli is a source of vitamins C and K. It also contains plenty of fiber, which helps fill you up, making it the perfect ingredient for a snack or lunchtime power bowl—1 cup contains about 30 calories and will satisfy your hunger. Broccoli has been linked to improved digestive and cardiovascular health and has wonderful, disease-preventing antioxidant properties. To make the most of its nutrients, eat it raw, or lightly steamed or sautéed.

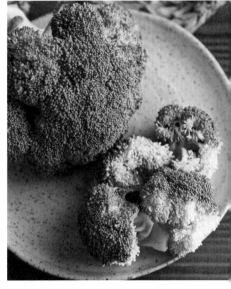

Broccoli

Carrots

Origin Afghanistan
Food Family Umbellifers
Nutrients Biotin, fiber, molybdenum, potassium, vitamins A, B6, C, K
Power Properties Crunchy and bright, carrots are a superfood loaded with nutrients, and are especially rich in antioxidants. They are full of vitamin A, which has been shown to improve eye health and prevent macular degeneration. Carrots add filling fiber, crunch, texture, and natural sweetness to a dish.

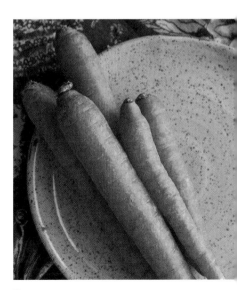

Carrots

Corn

Origin Mexico
Food Family Grasses
Nutrients Fiber, manganese, phosphorus, vitamins B3, B5, B6
Power Properties This bright yellow, juicy vegetable is a source of insoluble fiber and several antioxidants. Corn also provides starchy carbohydrates, which increase energy and fullness. You can use frozen, fresh, or canned corn. To use fresh corn, cook the cobs and then cut off the kernels, or just eat them right off the cob. Also, because corn is one of the more common genetically modified foods, be sure to buy organic, non-GMO varieties.

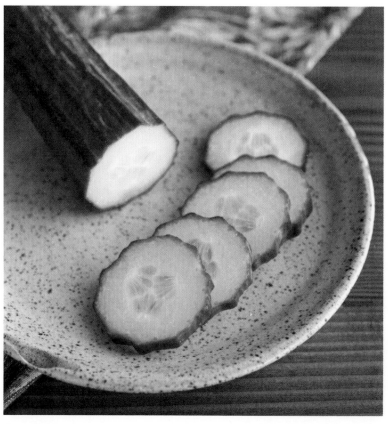

Cucumber

Cucumber

Origin India
Food Family Cucurbits
Nutrients Molybdenum, vitamins B5, K
Power Properties
Lean and green, cucumbers are a seriously healthy vegetable, loaded with unique phytonutrients that have antioxidant properties. They have also been shown to help reduce inflammation in the body. With a relatively low calorie content, they add bulk and volume to a meal, and fill you up without overloading on calories, making room for other ingredients to supply energy. Cucumbers come in several varieties, but the recipes in this book use English (greenhouse, seedless) cucumbers.

Garlic

Origin Middle Asia
Food Family Amaryllidaceae
Nutrients Copper, manganese, selenium, vitamins B6, C
Power Properties Because garlic is often used in small doses, it's not usually recommended for its vitamin and mineral content, but rather for its compounds, which include sulfur. Garlic has powerful antibacterial and antifungal properties, which help defend the body against illness. It has also been linked to improved cardiovascular health. It adds lots of flavor and immune-helping benefits to a dish.

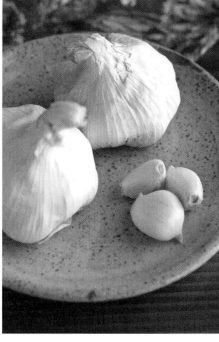

Garlic

Green Beans

Origin Peru
Food Family Legume
Nutrients Fiber, folate, manganese, vitamins C, K
Power Properties Green beans, also known as French beans, snap peas, or string beans, are a potent and tasty vegetable. They are rich in antioxidants and phytonutrients that improve immunity and cardiovascular heath. Because they also contain fiber, they are filling and help fuel the body, when paired with proteins and complex carbohydrates. Any variety of green beans will work well in power bowls, but try to use fresh instead of canned beans.

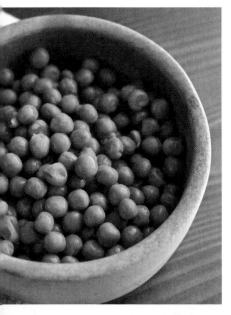

Green peas

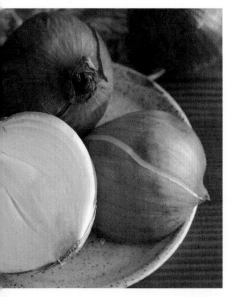

Onions

Green Peas

Origin India

Food Family Legume

Nutrients Copper, fiber, folate, manganese, phosphorus, protein, zinc, vitamins B, C, K

Power Properties These little gems are not to be underestimated. Not only are green peas full of vitamins, minerals, fiber, and proteins, they are also a source of carbohydrates that improve energy and stamina. Look for flash-frozen, organic, shelled green peas—simply thaw and use them. If you use canned green peas, buy an organic brand, free from preservatives or additives.

Mushrooms

Origin Believed to be North Africa

Food Family Fungi

Nutrients Copper, phosphorus, selenium, vitamins B2, B3, B5

Power Properties Edible mushrooms are incredibly flavorful, and can be found in many varieties, including wild, crimini, button, white, and portobello. All of these little fungi provide ample amounts of nutrients, including B vitamins and minerals. Mushrooms have also been shown to aid immune function.

Onion

Origin Believed to be Central Asia

Food Family Amaryllidaceae

Nutrients Biotin, copper, fiber, manganese, phosphorus, potassium, vitamins B6, C

Power Properties Onions, like garlic, are rich in sulfur-containing compounds, which makes them a great immune-boosting vegetable. They are a source of quercetin, an anti-inflammatory nutrient that has been shown to prevent and aid arthritic symptoms. Onions also help cardiovascular function. Use white or yellow onions, unless a recipe specifies a red onion, which is better consumed raw.

Radish

Origin Asia
Food Family Cabbage
Nutrients Fiber, folate, potassium, vitamin C
Power Properties One word comes to mind when thinking of radishes—spicy! While they are not spicy, like a hot pepper, they do have a "kick," making them an ideal addition to a power bowl, when you want a spicy flavor with added crunch. Not only do they taste unique, radishes are high in vitamin C and, therefore, have great antioxidant qualities. Radishes have also been shown to help regulate blood pressure, and support the respiratory system by relieving congestion and guarding the body against respiratory issues, like asthma and bronchitis. They come in several varieties but traditional red radishes and watermelon radishes are most common.

Red Cabbage

Origin Southern Europe
Food Family Cabbage
Nutrients Copper, fiber, manganese, potassium, vitamins B6, C, K
Power Properties This deep purple (more so than red) cabbage can be enjoyed in several ways: cooked, raw, stewed, and even pickled or fermented. It has been shown to stimulate cardiovascular health and digestive function, plus it has anti-inflammatory properties. Cabbage also contains the compound indole-3-carbinol, which is said to help with hormonal balance. It adds crunch, volume, and dietary fiber to a dish.

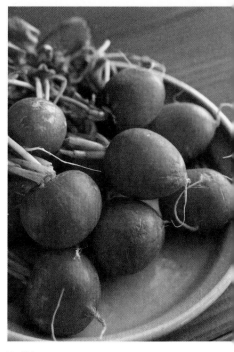

Radishes

Spinach

Origin Persia
Food Family Amaranthaceae
Nutrients Copper, folate, iron, magnesium, manganese, vitamins A, B, K
Power Properties Popeye didn't chow down on this dark, leafy green just for fun—he knew how powerful spinach is for strength and stamina! It is a nutrient-dense superfood that has a ton of vitamin K, which is an important nutrient for maintaining bone and skeletal health. Spinach is also a powerful anti-inflammatory and contains antioxidants to prevent pain and inflammation after a workout. If you're athletic, spinach should definitely be part of your diet.

Sprouts

Origin Various
Food Family Various
Nutrients Calcium, magnesium, vitamins A, C
Power Properties The term "sprouts" covers shoots from a wide variety of plants, including bean sprouts, alfalfa sprouts, and sunflower sprouts, which are often sold as a mixture. Not only are these little shoots rich in vitamins and minerals, they are also loaded with enzymes that help digestion. Sprouts also help reduce inflammation in the body. They make a great garnish, adding another little dose of nutrients and a shot of enzymes to improve the overall digestibility of a dish.

Sweet Potato

Origin Believed to be Egypt
Food Family Convolvulaceae
Nutrients Biotin, carbohydrates, copper, fiber, manganese, and vitamins A, B, C
Power Properties These brightly colored potatoes are rich in beta-carotenes, which give them their orange hue (although there are also some purple-colored varieties). Because of their vitamin and fiber content, as well as being a source of slow-releasing complex carbohydrates, sweet potatoes make an ideal

addition to a wake up power bowl to energize your body and keep you feeling full and satisfied all morning long.

Tomatoes and Sun-dried Tomatoes

Origin Andes region

Food Family Nightshade

Nutrients Biotin, copper, fiber, manganese, molybdenum, potassium, vitamins C, K

Power Properties Tomatoes are technically a fruit, but they are generally treated as a vegetable. Not only are they versatile, tomatoes are an amazing source of nutrients and carotenoids, including lycopene, which gives them their bright hue. Lycopene is a powerful antioxidant and has been associated with the reduced risk of disease and chronic health issues. Tomatoes come in many varieties and add flavor, bulk, antioxidants, and juiciness to a dish. Sun-dried tomatoes are simply tomatoes that have been dehydrated, using natural sunlight, and are typically preserved in jars of oil. They have the same nutrients as fresh tomatoes, with the added benefit of a concentrated taste.

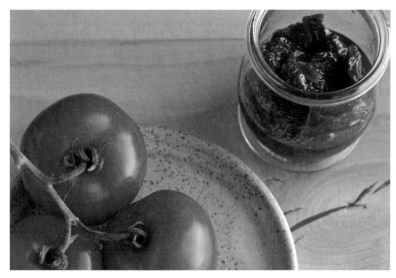

Tomatoes and sun-dried tomatoes

Ingredient Profiles:
Fruits

Bananas

Origin Malaysia and South Pacific

Food Family Banana

Nutrients Fiber, manganese, potassium, vitamins B6 and C

Power Properties Bananas are a fantastic source of nutrients for athletic activity and postexercise recovery. They help cardiovascular health, which is key for physical activity, as they contain potassium, which is essential for maintaining normal blood pressure and heart function. Also, the combination of vitamins, minerals, and low glycemic index complex carbohydrates makes bananas a prime choice for endurance athletes.

Cherries

Origin Asia

Food Family Prunus

Nutrients Carbohydrates, copper, fiber, manganese, potassium, vitamin C

Power Properties Cherries are sweet, juicy, and oh-so-satisfying, especially in the summer months, when they are in season. They meld wonderfully with sweeter flavors, and add a dose of antioxidants and fiber. Cherries are good for digestion and have been shown to help improve sleep, as they are naturally high in melatonin. You can use fresh, pitted cherries or frozen cherries, especially in the winter months, when you may not be able to find fresh cherries.

Dates

Origin Middle East

Food Family Palm tree

Nutrients Carbohydrates, copper, fiber, magnesium, manganese, potassium, vitamins B3, B5, B6

Power Properties Dates are an incredibly healthy food. As well as containing vitamins and minerals, these fruits boast lower glycemic

Dates

index carbohydrates, providing a boost of energy and lots of fiber to support digestive function. Use dried, pitted Medjool dates, or other dried pitted varieties, such as Deglet Noor or honey dates.

Goji Berries

Origin Asia
Food Family Nightshade
Nutrients Carbohydrates, copper, iron, selenium, vitamins A, B2
Power Properties These dried berries make a delicious power bowl addition before or after a workout, as their natural sugars will fuel the body with quick energy and replenish muscles after strenuous exercise. They also contain antioxidants and minerals to keep down inflammation, increase endurance, enhance stamina and strength, and promote cardiovascular health. When sprinkled on a power bowl, they add flavor and texture, too.

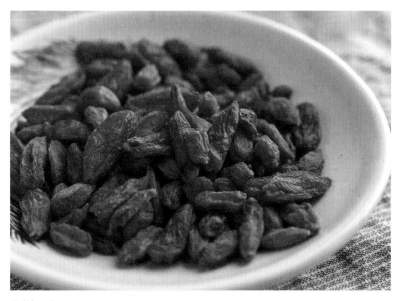

Goji berries

Grapefruit

Origin Caribbean
Food Family Rutaceae
Nutrients Biotin, carbohydrates, copper, fiber, potassium, vitamins A, B1, B5, C
Power Properties This sweet, tangy, and slightly sour citrus fruit is wonderfully nutritious. It provides the body with natural sugars for immediate energy, antioxidants, vitamins, minerals, and fiber. Like tomatoes, pink and red grapefruits also contain lycopene, which has been shown to combat disease. While grapefruits are naturally sweet, they also work in combination with savory ingredients, making them a great ingredient in a lunchtime or snack power bowl. For power bowls, any variety of grapefruit will work.

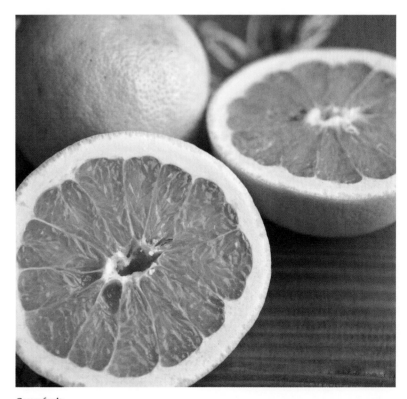

Grapefruit

Grapes

Origin Northern Iran
Food Family Vitis
Nutrients Carbohydrates, copper, vitamins B2, K
Power Properties This fruit belongs to the berry family and adds sweetness, juiciness, texture, and vitamins to a dish. Grapes come in many varieties. For power bowls, use red or green seedless varieties. Not only do they make a great addition to sweeter power bowls, grapes also work well with savory ingredients, which is why they make the perfect addition to a Waldorf-salad inspired power bowl (see page 126).

Kiwi

Origin China
Food Family Nightshade
Nutrients Carbohydrates, copper, fiber, potassium, vitamins C, E, K
Power Properties This green fruit really packs a punch. Just one kiwifruit has 85 percent of the daily recommended dietary allowance of vitamin C, so it's definitely an antioxidant-rich immune booster. Kiwi are also rich in potassium, and have been linked to improved cardiovascular health. These sweet and slightly tart fruits provide antioxidants, fiber, and natural sugars for immediate energy. While the skin is edible, it's recommended to remove it before eating.

Lemons

Origin Northeast India, Burma, and China
Food Family Rutaceae
Nutrients Vitamin C
Power Properties These tangy citrus fruits are vitamin C bombs. They provide ample amounts of antioxidants, as well, and have been shown to stimulate the production of digestive enzymes. The zest and oil of lemons can be used as well as the juice.

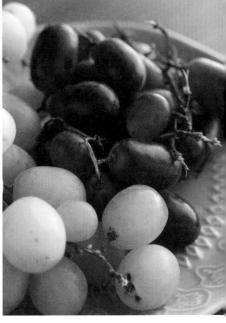

Grapes

Limes

Origin Thought to be Southeast Asia
Food Family Citrus
Nutrients Carbohydrates, folate, vitamin C
Power Properties Like lemons, these bright green citrus fruits are loaded with Vitamin C. The citrus tang from limes works in sweet and savory dishes, livening up the flavors. Like lemons, you can use the zest, oil, and juice of a lime.

Mango

Origin South Asia
Food Family Mangifera
Nutrients Carbohydrates, copper, fiber, potassium, vitamins A, B6, C, E, K
Power Properties Rich in fiber and loaded with antioxidant-rich vitamins, mangoes are a fruit to contend with. While they may not be the easiest to peel, once the skin is removed the rewards are plenty. Mangoes are naturally sweet, provide carbohydrates, and are naturally low on the glycemic index, meaning that they don't spike blood-sugar levels. Their fiber helps to slow the release of the fruit's natural sugars into the bloodstream, and helps digestion.

Orange

Origin South Asia, China, and India
Food Family Citrus
Nutrients Calcium, carbohydrates, copper, fiber, folate, potassium, vitamins B1, B5, C
Power Properties Oranges are superhydrating, sweet, healthy, and satisfying. These bright citrus fruits are loaded with vitamin C, B vitamins, fiber, and minerals. Their color comes from the antioxidant carotenoids they contain. Oranges are known for their immune-boosting functions, and help the body to combat the negative effects of stress by supporting the adrenal glands.

Mangoes

Peach

Origin China
Food Family Rosaceae
Nutrients Carbohydrates, fiber, potassium, vitamins A, B3, C
Power Properties These versatile, soft, and sweet stone fruits are perfect in sweet and savory dishes. You can enjoy peaches raw, stewed, baked, and even grilled. They add vitamins and minerals, along with digestion-boosting fiber to help you to feel full.

Pineapple

Origin South America
Food Family Bromeliads
Nutrients Carbohydrates, copper, manganese, vitamins B1, B6, C
Power Properties After a good, resistance-training workout, the body needs usable sugar for quick energy. Pineapples contain plenty of natural sugar, increase energy quickly, and refuel tired muscles. Along with the workout benefits, pineapples have a natural enzyme called "bromelain" to help digestion, are rich in antioxidants, and have anti-inflammatory properties, which make them ideal for preventing postworkout inflammation.

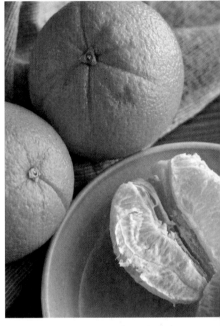

Oranges

Raisins

Origin Middle East
Food Family Vitis
Nutrients Carbohydrates, copper, fiber, manganese, potassium, vitamins B1, B2, B6
Power Properties A raisin may simply be a dried grape, but it has a different nutrient profile compared to the fresh fruit. Raisins contain dietary fiber to improve digestive function, minerals, and vitamins —particularly B vitamins. They are slightly higher on the glycemic index than grapes, but enjoyed in smaller doses they provide immediate energy and keep digestion running smoothly. Used as a garnish, raisins add nutrients, carbohydrates, and fiber. When buying raisins, look for ones without added sulfur dioxide.

Ingredient Profiles:
Sweeteners

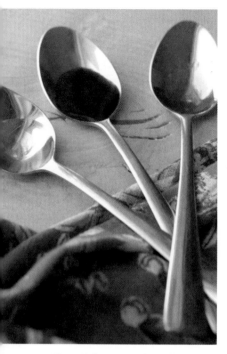

Almond, lemon, and vanilla extracts

Almond, Lemon, and Vanilla Extracts

Origin Various
Food Family Various
Nutrients N/A
Power Properties While these extracts do not bring any significant nutritional benefit, just a few drops add loads of zest to complement other ingredients in a dish. They are made by extracting the flavor of the source ingredient, and adding it to a liquid base, which is often alcohol. These potent extracts create bursts of deliciousness. Always buy "pure" extracts with no artificial or imitation flavors.

Brown Rice Syrup

Origin Asia
Food Family Grasses
Nutrients Calcium, carbohydrates
Power Properties In ancient times, rice syrup was believed to be of divine origin, and it's no wonder, because the taste of this sweet, sticky syrup is out of this world. Brown rice syrup is sourced from a whole grain and is unrefined, which makes it a healthier alternative, compared to regular sugar, as it doesn't have the same addictive properties. Thanks to its liquid consistency, it's a great way to drizzle some natural sweetness into a dish. Like any natural sugar, use it in moderation, as it is high on the glycemic index.

Coconut Nectar

Origin Southeast Asia
Food Family Palm tree
Nutrients Amino acids, carbohydrates
Power Properties This sweet, sticky nectar is made from the sap of coconut palm tree flower blossoms. It is much lower on the glycemic index than table sugar, making it a natural sweetener that, when

consumed in moderation, won't spike blood sugar levels. A total of 17 amino acids and some trace minerals are found in raw coconut nectar, which is another reason why it's superior to refined sugar.

Coconut Palm Sugar

Origin Southeast Asia
Food Family Palm tree
Nutrients Carbohydrates
Power Properties Coconut palm sugar is a granulated, natural sweetner produced from coconut palm trees. It has a subtle sweetness and makes a fantastic garnish to amp flavor. It is low on the glycemic index, making it an alternative to sugar that won't spike blood sugar, when consumed in moderation.

Pure Maple Syrup

Origin North America
Food Family Maple tree
Nutrients Calcium, carbohydrates, iron, magnesium, manganese, potassium, zinc
Power Properties This dark, sweet syrup is produced from the sap of the maple tree, and adds a little sweetness, along with health-enhancing minerals, to a dish. This syrup is also lower than sugar on the glycemic index, making it a great alternative sweetener. As a natural sweetener, it releases energy into the bloodstream more slowly, preventing spikes in blood-sugar levels. If possible, use a Grade A maple syrup, which can be purchased at most grocery stores. It is important to buy a pure graded maple syrup and avoid imitation maple syrups.

Ingredient Profiles:
Herbs & Spices

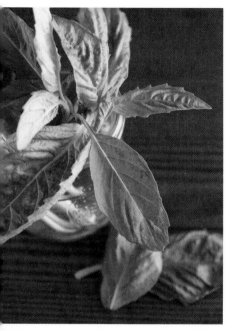

Basil

Basil

Origin Believed to be India
Food Family Lamiaceae
Nutrients Copper, manganese, vitamins A, C, K
Power Properties Basil is called the "king of herbs" or the "royal herb." It is so aromatic, it's almost impossible to miss it when it is added to a dish. Basil is also a good source of vitamin K, along with other minerals and vitamins. It has been shown to prevent unhealthy bacterial growth in the body. As well as being a natural "antibacterial," it is also known to have anti-inflammatory effects and promote cardiovascular health. Use regular and Thai basil for their flavor, nutrients, and powerful health benefits. Unless otherwise indicated, use fresh basil rather than dried.

Cayenne

Origin South America
Food Family Nightshade
Nutrients Fiber, manganese, vitamins B6, C, E, K
Power Properties Cayenne peppers, which are the source of ground cayenne, have similar merits to red pepper flakes and chili powder (see page 48). The pepper contains the nutritional compound capsacin, which has been shown to be an effective treatment for pain associated with arthritis, because of its natural anti-inflammatory properties. The power properties of this spice come from its thermogenic abilities, which promote fat-burning in the body and, along with regular exercise, can help with weight loss.

Cilantro

Origin Europe, North Africa, and Asia
Food Family Umbellifers
Nutrients Vitamins A, C, K
Power Properties Cilantro is a relative of parsley and has a potent flavor. Because of its unique taste it isn't loved by everyone. So, if you aren't a huge fan, omit it from the recipe. This fresh and citrusy herb is rich in vitamins, and has been shown to help with blood-sugar stabilization and manage healthy cholesterol levels, plus it has antioxidant properties. Cilantro adds vitamins to a dish and a flavor that melds wonderfully with ingredients, such as limes and coconut. Unless otherwise indicated, use fresh cilantro leaves instead of dried.

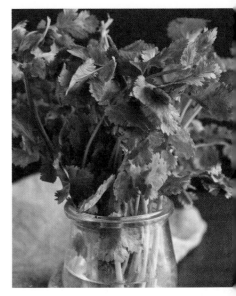

Cilantro

Cinnamon

Origin India
Food Family Lauraceae
Nutrients Calcium, fiber, manganese
Power Properties This rich, aromatic spice is incredibly flavorful, and works well in both sweet and savory dishes. It offers many powerful health benefits, including blood-sugar stabilization, cardiovascular advantages, and has natural antibacterial and antifungal properties. Use cinnamon in breakfast bowls, as it is also known to naturally stimulate the metabolism, and treat bowls, as it complements naturally sweet ingredients, such as apples. You can find cinnamon in whole sticks or ground. For these recipes, use ground cinnamon.

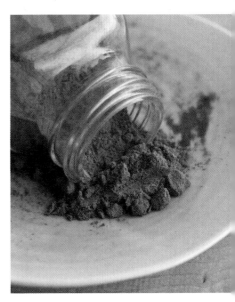

Cinnamon

Cumin

Origin Egypt, India and Eastern Mediterranean
Food Family Umbellifers
Nutrients Calcium, copper, iron, magnesium, manganese
Power Properties Cumin has a distinct tang that works well in spicy dishes, and is often used in Mexican- and Indian-inspired food. It contains iron, and has been shown to improve energy levels and immunity. It is sold as whole or ground seeds. In these recipes, use ground cumin, as the flavor is slightly more potent.

Dill

Origin Russia, Mediterranean, and Western Africa
Food Family Apiaceae
Nutrients Manganese, vitamin C
Power Properties Dill enhances the taste of many dishes and, along with adding small amounts of vitamin C and manganese, it has been shown to have antibacterial properties and antioxidant power. It works well with ingredients, such as salmon and lemon, and it always adds a touch of freshness. Unless otherwise indicated, use fresh dill rather than dried.

Kaffir Lime Leaves

Origin Asia
Food Family Rutaceae
Nutrients N/A
Power Properties Kaffir lime leaves come from the Kaffir lime plant and are used in Southeast Asian cooking. The leaf provides an incredible aromatic and astringent note. While it doesn't necessarily provide any significant nutrients, the leaf has been traditionally used to improve dental health—by brushing it over the teeth—and its essential oils are also believed to have a positive effect on the mind and body by creating energy and positivity.

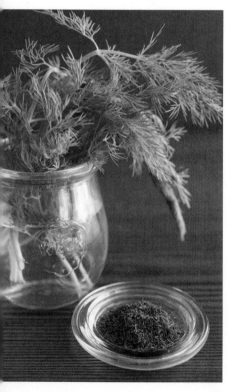

Dill

Mint

Origin Various
Food Family Lamiaceae
Nutrients Calcium, magnesium, phosphorus, potassium, vitamin C
Power Properties This versatile herb makes its way into both sweet and savory dishes and beverages. Mint is wonderfully refreshing and makes a great power bowl garnish. Not only does it add small amounts of nutrients, including minerals and vitamin C, it has a high antioxidant capacity and has been shown to assist digestion, immunity, and oral health. In these recipes, use sprigs of fresh mint leaves for the best flavor and nutritional bonus.

Nutmeg

Origin Indonesia
Food Family Myristicaceae
Nutrients Calcium, fiber, iron, magnesium, vitamin B6
Power Properties Nutmeg has a rich, aromatic, and comforting aroma, and is commonly paired with cinnamon. Not only does this spice make a lovely addition to power bowls, it also contains fiber, minerals, and vitamins. Nutmeg has also been shown to have anti-inflammatory properties, enhance digestive function, and help with circulation.

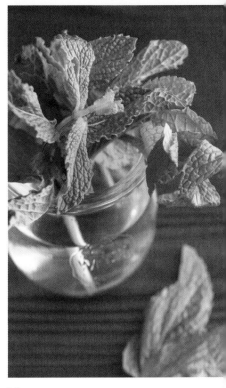

Mint

Paprika

Origin Central Mexico
Food Family Nightshade
Nutrients Fiber, iron, magnesium, vitamins A, B6, E
Power Properties Like chili powder and cayenne, paprika is another spice that originates from peppers. It adds spice and aroma, and a little goes a long way. It also contains vitamin A, thanks to its natural carotenoids, which are known to improve eye health and prevent macular degeneration. Paprika also has vitamins, minerals, and fiber, as well as the nutritional compound capsacin, which encourages fat-burning and prevents inflammation.

Parsley

Origin Mediterranean
Food Family Apiaceae
Nutrients Copper, folate, iron, vitamins A, C, K
Power Properties Parsley is a wonderful health-boosting herb. Its subtle flavor makes it popular with most people. It provides copious amounts of antioxidants, and has been shown to improve cardiovascular health and protect against arthritic diseases. This leafy herb is loaded with vitamin K—in fact, just 1/2 cup of chopped parsley contains over 500 percent of the daily recommended dietary allowance! In these recipes, use fresh parsley instead of dried.

Red Pepper Flakes/Chili Powder

Origin Mexico
Food Family Nightshade
Nutrients Copper, fiber, vitamins A, B6, E, K
Power Properties These flakes are made from hot red peppers, which have been dried and crushed. They have a nutritional compound called capsacin, which is a natural anti-inflammatory, and has been studied as an effective treatment for the pain associated with arthritis. This compound can also help with postworkout inflammation. The pepper's thermogenic properties, which aid fat-burning in the body, can help promote weight loss, along with regular exercise. These recipes use both red pepper flakes (also called chili flakes) and ground chili powder.

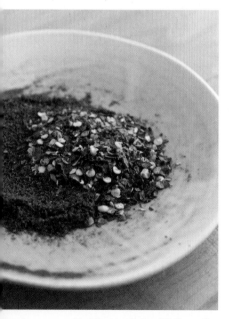

Red Pepper flakes/Chili powder

Taco Seasoning

Origin Mexico
Food Family N/A
Nutrients N/A
Power Properties In this book, some recipes call for a spice blend that's often called "taco seasoning," as the blend of spices works wonderfully with Mexican-inspired dishes. Most often, taco seasoning is a blend of chili, garlic, onion powder, cumin, cayenne, paprika, and salt. While there are many variations, the general taste is consistent. You can use any brand of taco seasoning, or make your own blend. When you buy taco seasoning, make sure that it has no added sugar, MSG, or artificial ingredients.

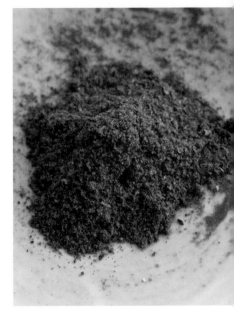

Taco seasoning

Thyme

Origin Southern Europe
Food Family Lamiaceae
Nutrients Iron, manganese, vitamin C
Power Properties Thyme is a savory, comforting herb that adds a subtle flavor to many dishes. It has been used in traditional medicine for many ailments, and has been shown to help guard against chest and respiratory problems, such as coughs, bronchitis, and chest congestion. This herb also contains a small amount of vitamin C, iron, and manganese. You can use dried or fresh thyme.

Turmeric

Origin Southern India
Food Family Zingiberaceae
Nutrients Copper, fiber, iron, manganese, potassium, vitamin B6
Power Properties This bright yellow spice has returned to the spotlight in recent years as a superfood. Research has found that this potent spice has anti-inflammatory benefits, helps to decrease the risk of cancer, encourages detoxification in the body, and improves cognitive function. It also helps with blood-sugar balance and kidney function, and helps relieve certain kinds of arthritis and digestive disorders.

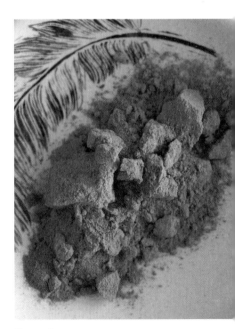

Turmeric

Essential Tools

To make power bowls you will need some general kitchen tools. You may already have most of them. However, you may also be ready to make some upgrades.

High-speed Blender

The base of many of the power bowls in this book is a combination of ingredients that have been blended together. Ideally, you need a high-speed blender, which will create a smooth, creamy, mixture with no grittiness.

Serving Bowls

You can't make power bowls without a selection of bowls to serve them in. You will need a few smaller snack bowls for dessert-sized portions; a couple of medium-sized bowls for breakfast and lunch; some deeper, soup or salad bowls, that can also hold smoothie mixtures; plus some larger bowls for meal-sized power bowls.

Large Skillet or Frying Pan

Many of the meal-sized bowls are made on the stovetop, so having a large skillet or frying pan, or a shallow (2.5 quart) saucepan, is key. Use a pan that is about 13 inches in diameter and made with nontoxic materials, such as cast iron, stainless steel, or ceramic.

Set of Knives

Making power bowls involves a lot of chopping. A set of good quality knives is helpful, as you'll likely enjoy the process of cutting, slicing, and dicing a little more with the ease of a good knife.

Measuring Cups and Spoons

While you won't often be weighing ingredients on a food scale, you will need a set of measuring spoons and cups.

Techniques

Making power bowls requires some simple techniques that will enable you to preserve the minerals and other benefits of the ingredients, as well as their textures and flavors.

Sautéing

For many of the meal bowls in this book, you will sauté the ingredients in a skillet, frying pan, or shallow saucepan to cook either the whole dish or portions of it. The ingredients are browned and cooked, while preserving their texture, moisture, and flavor, which is very important for power bowls, as each ingredient is meant to stand out. Usually, I recommend using oil, such as olive or coconut, to prevent the ingredients from sticking to the pan. One important thing to note when sautéing is not to overheat the pan, as this can cause ingredients to stick and burn. Using medium to high heat at first, and then lowering the heat to low to medium, near the end of cooking, is best. It is important to note that certain oils should not be used for sautéing, because they have a low smoke point and can turn rancid at higher heats; this includes flax, walnut, safflower, and sunflower oils.

Baking

While my aim was to make most of the recipes in power bowls bake-free, there are a few recipes that require this method, mostly for potatoes and some proteins. To bake them, use a large baking pan lined with parchment paper. This works wonderfully when baking potatoes, as they can be spread evenly over the pan without any risk of sticking or burning, and the cleanup is a dream. If you are baking a protein such as salmon, chicken, or turkey, use an ovenproof baking dish with a lid, as this will lock in the moisture and flavor, leaving you with a delicious protein that is not dried out or overcooked. For baking, temperatures are given in degrees Fahrenheit. However, if you need degrees Celsius, refer to the conversion chart on page 185.

Blending

Many of the power bowls in this book have a smooth and nutritious "base" that is created by blending ingredients together, using a high-speed blender (see Tools, page 50). It's important to practice this technique to get the best consistency. Combine the ingredients in the blender and use a low speed to break up most of the pieces. After about 10 seconds, slowly increase the speed and, if necessary, use a tamper to keep the ingredients blending smoothly. It is sometimes helpful to stop the blender, give it a little shake, then blend again to keep the ingredients moving through. After about 30 seconds, increase the speed to the highest level and blend for 10 to 20 seconds, until the mixture is completely smooth.

Layering and Arranging Ingredients

Power bowls are all about the melding of power-giving ingredients that supply different tastes, textures, and nutrient combinations. But one especially enjoyable aspect of making a delicious power bowl is presentation. Most of the recipes in this book have many components, and the arranging or layering of each ingredient gives the bowls their bright, colorful, and appetizing appearance, and makes each bite an exciting discovery of tastes and textures. If you are in a hurry, there's no harm in tossing the ingredients into the bowl and digging in, but it is worth taking an extra minute or two to layer the ingredients in a beautiful arrangement that showcases each color and texture. Not only does appealing food cause us to salivate (which improves digestion), it gives us more appreciation for the food we are about to enjoy, and we take a little more time enjoying each bite (which also helps digestion). To layer the ingredients, place the bulkier items at the bottom of the bowl, as the base. This includes complex carbohydrates (oats, rice, quinoa, beans, potatoes, etc.) or a smoothie mixture. Arrange the smaller portions of colorful and textured ingredients, such as berries and other fruits, nuts, seeds, and garnishes in sections on top. This gives the power bowls depth, beauty, and, of course, makes each bite different from the last.

Special Diets

Grain-Free
Grains have been linked to inflammatory diseases and disorders, and individuals with diseases, such as Crohn's, have benefited from eliminating all grains—the seeds of grasslike plants, such as wheat, corn, oats, and rice—from their diets. If a recipe contains grains, a swap can be made. For example, substitute rice with sweet potatoes or black beans.

Peanut-Free/Nut-Free
Many of the recipes are peanut- and nut-free. However, where nuts are used, simply omit them. If a recipe calls for a nutbased milk, such as almond, substitute a nonnut milk such as rice, soy, or coconut.

Palaeolithic
The Palaeolithic (or "paleo") diet is based on the foods consumed by early humans, mostly meat, fish, vegetables, and fruit. Many of the recipes in this book would be suitable for this diet, with the omission of any grain and dairy ingredients. Replace the grains with a complex carbohydrate, such as sweet potato, to maintain the nutritional balance of the bowl.

Pregnancy
I was pregnant during the making of this book, so it is safe to say that all of the recipes are suitable during pregnancy, as long as your doctor has not made any specific dietary recommendations. Many of the recipes in this book are high in the nutrients that are vital during pregnancy.

Diabetes/Low-Glycemic Diet
A diet recommended for diabetics, also known as a low-glycemic diet, focuses on foods that do not have a great impact on glucose levels in the body. Diabetics, or individuals who are following a low glycemic diet, should be mindful of the amount of sugar in food. Many of the recipes in this book are low in sugar and contain low glycemic foods. Others are higher in naturally occurring sugars from fruits and other whole foods, and these are generally lower on the glycemic index. Anyone following this diet should be mindful of any foods they know they should avoid.

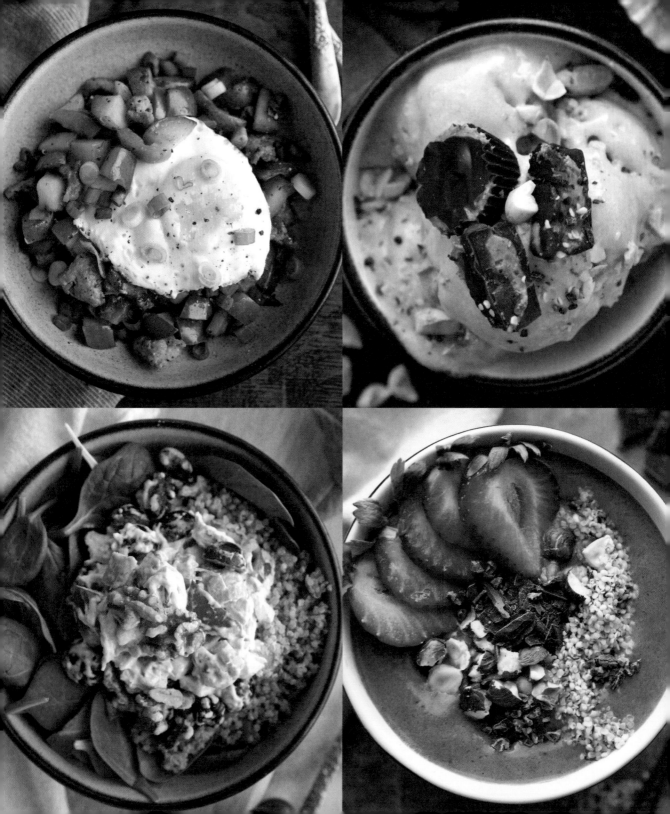

PART TWO

Power Bowl Recipes

These meals and snacks will give you all the nutrition you need, whether you've got a busy day at work or you're training for a marathon. There are large bowls to fill you up, workout bowls to boost your energy, and treat bowls to enjoy when you need a little something special.

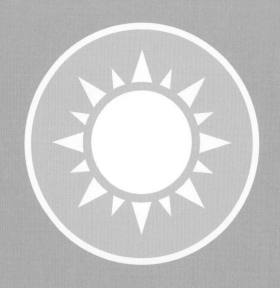

Wake Up Bowls

Start the day with a bowl that supplies sustained energy from proteins and complex carbohydrates, fiber to aid digestion, and plenty of vitamins and minerals to support your body. Some can be prepared in minutes —or overnight—for a quick start to the day; others take more time and are perfect for a leisurely weekend brunch.

Active Ingredients

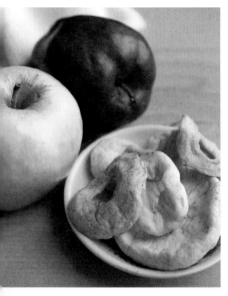

Apples and dried apples

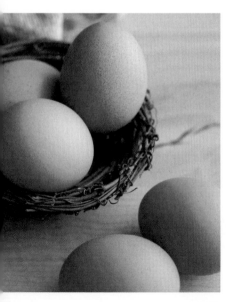

Eggs

Apples & Dried Apples
Origin Central Asia
Food Family Rosaceae
Nutrients Carbohydrates, fiber, vitamin C
Power Properties Apples are a fantastic source of dietary fiber and vitamin C. Fiber promotes digestion and keeps your body feeling sustained, while vitamin C supports the adrenal glands that help to regulate stress hormones and keep energy levels stable. Choose dried apples that do not contain added sweeteners or sulfates.

Chia Seeds
Origin Mayan and Aztec regions
Food Family Lamiaceae
Nutrients Calcium, fiber, manganese, omega fatty acids, phosphorus, and zinc
Power Properties Chia means "strength" and this mighty seed is rich in digestive-enhancing fiber and healthy fats that will satisfy the body for hours. Chia seeds are available in white or black varieties, and both offer a raft of nutritional benefits.

Eggs
Origin South East Asia and India
Food Family Animal
Nutrients Biotin, choline, fats, protein, selenium, vitamins B2 and B12
Power Properties It's no wonder that eggs are thought of as a staple breakfast food: They are high in protein and fats, and help to keep blood-sugar levels stable. Both the white and yolk contain protein, and the yolks of pasture-raised eggs are a source of nutrients and omega-3 fats. Choose organic pasture-raised or "free-range" eggs, as these have been produced in the most ethical manner and have the highest level of nutrients.

Granola

Origin First produced in the United States

Food Family N/A

Nutrients Calcium, carbohydrates, fiber, iron, magnesium, protein, B vitamins

Power Properties Granola is a mixture of whole grains, such as rolled oats, grain flakes, and puffed grains; a sweetener such as honey; nuts; and seeds. It is an ideal breakfast option, as it is rich in complex carbohydrates, protein, and healthy fats. Choose one that is free from artificial additives, is naturally sweetened, and has less than 6g of sugar per ¼-cup serving. You can also make your own.

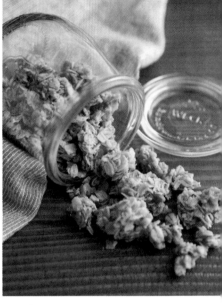

Granola

Oats, Rolled

Origin Middle East

Food Family Grasses

Nutrients Carbohydrates, fiber, iron, magnesium, B vitamins

Power Properties This whole grain is bursting with nutrients and slow-releasing, complex carbohydrates. Always look for plain, unsweetened rolled oats. Oats can be contaminated with gluten, so if you have an allergy or intolerance look for "certified" gluten-free oats.

Puffed Brown Rice Cereal & Other Puffed Grains

Origin Asia and others

Food Family Oryza and others

Nutrients Carbohydrates, copper, fiber, iron, manganese, selenium, B vitamins

Power Properties These "puffed" grains have been steamed to add moisture. Then they are heated until they pop like popcorn. Puffed brown rice is a nutritious whole grain that provides fiber and helps sustain long-lasting energy. Other puffed whole grains include amaranth, wheat, buckwheat, and quinoa, which have the same properties. Choose plain versions that are free from added sweeteners.

Nutty Quinoa Porridge

SERVES · 4
PREPARATION TIME · 2 MINUTES
COOKING TIME · 8 MINUTES

1½ cups unsweetened almond milk
3 tablespoons natural almond butter
2 tablespoons coconut palm sugar
2 cups cooked quinoa
½ cup fresh raspberries
¼ cup diced or slivered almonds
¼ cup toasted coconut flakes

Waking up to a warm, filling bowl of naturally sweet porridge is an appealing thought on any morning. This nutty quinoa porridge takes it up a notch by incorporating creamy almond butter and almond milk, as well as low-glycemic coconut palm sugar, and protein-rich quinoa for long-lasting energy.

1 Combine the almond milk and almond butter in a small saucepan, set over medium heat, and cook for 3 minutes, until the nut butter melts into the almond milk, and stir until the mixture is smooth.

2 Stir in the coconut palm sugar.

3 Add in the cooked quinoa and stir for 3–4 minutes to incorporate with the almond milk mixture and heat through.

4 Divide the quinoa porridge equally among four bowls and top the bowls with the raspberries, almonds, and toasted coconut. Serve immediately.

> **Try this!**
> ## Pumpkin Spice Quinoa Porridge
> Pumpkin is a powerful superfood, filled with beta-carotene, antioxidants, and fiber. Add the delightful flavor of pumpkin pie to this recipe by adding ¼ cup of pure pumpkin puree with the quinoa, along with ½ teaspoon of pumpkin pie spice. Swap out the ½ cup fresh raspberries and amp up the Fall inspiration by using ½ cup diced apple and an extra pinch of cinnamon to top each bowl.

PER SERVING	
Calories	341
Protein	10g
Fat	22g
Carbohydrate	34g
Sugar	7g
Dietary fiber	9g
Vitamins	all B vitamins
Minerals	calcium, iron

Made 6/22/20 - very good! I halved the recipe and used regular milk, cinnamon almond butter, regular (not slivered) almonds, and strawberries instead of raspberries. Would make again!

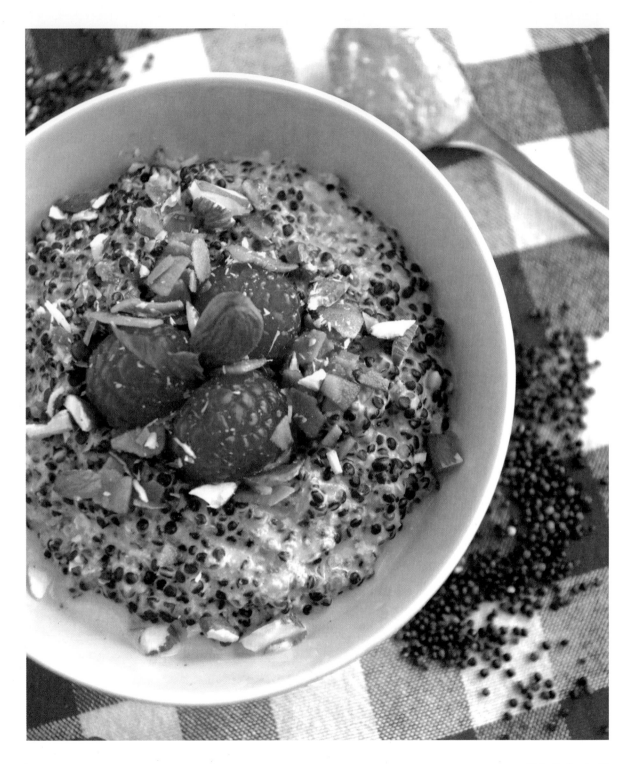

Try this!

Blueberry, Maple & Quinoa Porridge

Increase the fruit content of the quinoa porridge by using fresh
blueberries, which burst with antioxidants. Adding maple syrup,
a natural, unrefined sweetener, enhances the delicious taste.

SERVES · 4
PREPARATION TIME · 2 MINUTES
COOKING TIME · 8 MINUTES

1½ cups unsweetened almond milk
3 tablespoons natural almond butter
1 tablespoon pure maple syrup
2 cups cooked quinoa
¾ cup fresh blueberries
¼ cup chopped or slivered almonds
¼ cup toasted coconut flakes

1 Combine the almond milk and almond butter in a small
saucepan, set over medium heat, and cook for 3 minutes,
until the nut butter melts into the almond milk, and stir
until the mixture is smooth.

2 Stir in the pure maple syrup.

3 Add in the cooked quinoa and ¼ cup of the blueberries, and
stir for 3–4 minutes to incorporate with the almond milk mixture
and heat through.

4 Divide quinoa porridge equally among four bowls and top the
bowls with the remaining blueberries, almonds, and toasted
coconut. Serve immediately.

Hemp, Golden Berry & Coconut

SERVES · 2
PREPARATION TIME · 10 MINUTES

1¹/2 cups plain coconut yogurt
¹/2 cup gluten-free puffed grain cereal (brown rice, millet, or sorghum)
2 tablespoons raw hempseeds
¹/2 cup dried golden berries
1 medium banana, sliced
¹/2 cup fresh blueberries
1 tablespoon raw honey
1 tablespoon natural almond butter

This tasty wake up bowl contains plenty of protein, thanks to the hempseeds, as well as healthy fats and fiber from the yogurt and almond butter. There's also crunch and complex carbohydrates from the puffed rice cereal, and vitamins and antioxidants from the golden berries and other fruits.

1 Divide the coconut yogurt between two bowls.

2 Top the yogurt with the puffed grain cereal, hempseeds, golden berries, sliced banana, and blueberries. Drizzle raw honey and almond butter over each bowl. Serve immediately.

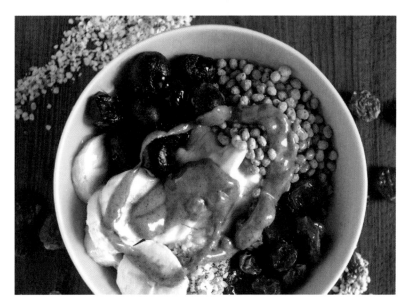

PER SERVING	
Calories	327
Protein	8g
Fat	15g
Carbohydrate	45g
Sugar	22g
Dietary fiber	6g
Vitamins	B
Minerals	iron, magnesium

Try this!
Hemp & Mixed Berry Greek Yogurt

Replace the golden berries with an equal amount of mixed dried cranberries, blueberries, and mulberries, which are all rich in antioxidants. Increase the protein content of this bowl by using 1¹/2 cups full-fat plain Greek yogurt in place of the coconut yogurt.

Super Chia Muesli

SERVES · 2
PREPARATION TIME · 5 MINUTES
COOKING TIME · 60 MINUTES

FOR THE LEMON CHIA PUDDING
4 tablespoons chia seeds
1 cup unsweetened almond milk
1 tablespoon fresh lemon zest
1 tablespoon raw honey

FOR THE TOPPING
10 raw almonds, chopped
5 raw pecans, chopped
1/2 cup mixed fresh berries
4 dried apricots, chopped
2 tablespoons shredded unsweetened
   coconut
1 tablespoon 70% dark chocolate shavings
1 tablespoon fresh lemon zest

This bowl is sure to bring some punch and brightness to your day. Lemon zest and chia seeds wake up the digestive system, while pecans and almonds add protein and omega-rich fats. The berries, apricots, and dark chocolate shavings bring sweetness and antioxidants.

1 To make the lemon chia pudding, combine the chia seeds, almond milk, lemon zest, and honey in an 8-ounce jar or a small airtight container. Seal and shake vigorously for 10 seconds. Chill in the refrigerator for 30 minutes, then remove and shake for 10 seconds again. Return to the refrigerator for another 30 minutes, or leave in the refrigerator overnight.

2 Divide the chia pudding between two bowls. Top the bowls with the chopped almonds and pecans, mixed berries, chopped dried apricots, shredded unsweetened coconut, dark chocolate shavings, and lemon zest. Serve immediately.

Try this!
Loaded Chocolate Chia Muesli

Dark chocolate tastes delicious, but it's also full of antioxidants, and this power bowl will make a fantastic breakfast or brunch treat. To make a chocolate chia pudding, replace the lemon zest in the pudding with 1 tablespoon of unsweetened cocoa powder. Prepare the bowl as directed, but replace the lemon zest in the topping with an extra tablespoon of 70% dark chocolate shavings.

PER SERVING	
Calories	329
Protein	6g
Fat	18g
Carbohydrate	25g
Sugar	16g
Dietary fiber	7g
Vitamins	A, C
Minerals	calcium, iron, magnesium

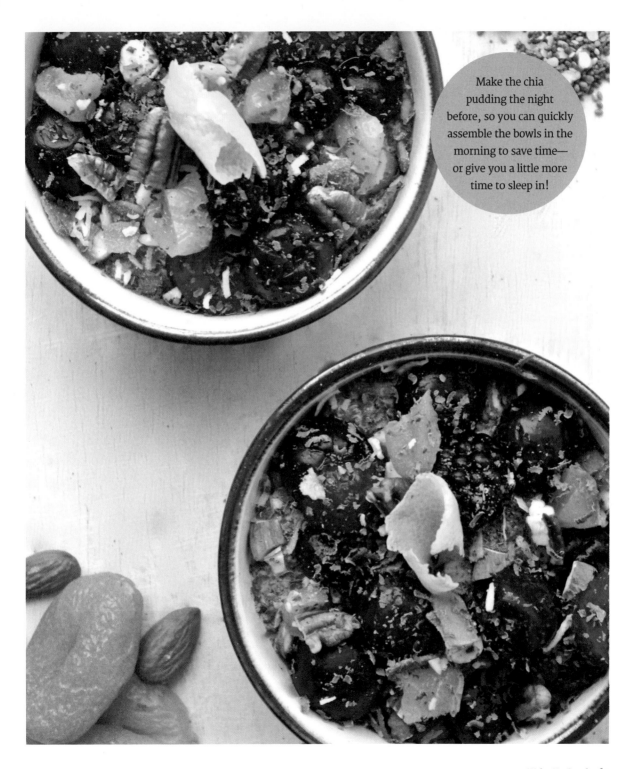

Make the chia pudding the night before, so you can quickly assemble the bowls in the morning to save time— or give you a little more time to sleep in!

PB & J Overnight Oats

SERVES · 1
PREPARATION TIME · 10 MINUTES
COOKING TIME · 5 HOURS

FOR THE OVERNIGHT OAT BASE
1/2 cup rolled oats
1 cup unsweetened almond milk
1 tablespoon chia seeds
1 teaspoon honey
1/2 tablespoon natural peanut butter

FOR THE TOPPING
1 tablespoon natural strawberry or raspberry
   jelly or jam
3 sliced strawberries
6 fresh raspberries
1/2 tablespoon natural peanut butter
1 tablespoon crushed peanuts

Never underestimate the classic combination of peanut butter and jelly—sweet and nutty, it is a match made in heaven. Overnight oats are the perfect breakfast on a busy morning, as they are rich in healthy fats, fiber, and carbohydrates. This bowl will fill you up faster than you can say "PB & J!"

1 To make the overnight oat base, combine the rolled oats, almond milk, chia seeds, honey, and 1/2 tablespoon peanut butter in a bowl. Stir to combine, making sure the honey and peanut butter are incorporated with the other ingredients.

2 Cover the bowl with plastic wrap or a lid and chill for at least 5 hours, or overnight. As they soak, the oats and chia will absorb the liquid until they attain the consistency of cooked oatmeal.

3 When the oats are fully soaked, transfer them to a serving bowl. Top the oat mixture with the jelly or jam, and berries. Drizzle with the 1/2 tablespoon natural peanut butter and finish with the crushed peanuts. Serve immediately.

PER SERVING	
Calories	437
Protein	13g
Fat	17g
Carbohydrate	58g
Sugar	20g
Dietary fiber	13g
Vitamins	B
Minerals	calcium, iron, magnesium

Try this!
Blackberry, Maple & Flax Overnight Oats

Blackberries are a wonderful source of antioxidants, vitamin C, and fiber, and they taste amazing alongside calcium-rich maple syrup in this tasty recipe. The flaxseed contains ample amounts of fiber to fill you up and fuel you through the morning. Omit the peanut butter from the oat base, and replace the chai seeds and honey with 1 tablespoon of ground flaxseeds and 1 teaspoon of pure maple syrup. Once the oat base is ready, replace all of the toppings with 1/4 cup fresh blackberries and drizzle them with 1 teaspoon pure maple syrup.

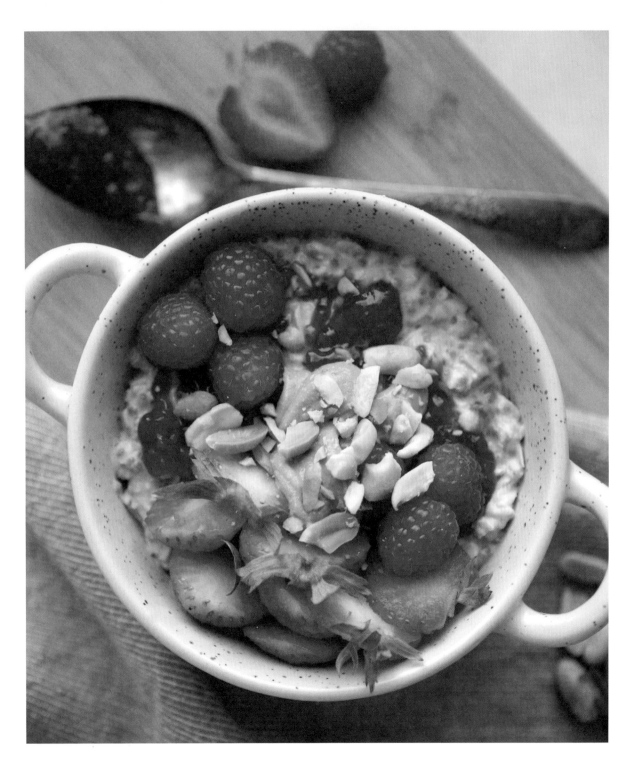

Try this!

Creamy Cashew & Coconut Overnight Oats

If you have a jam-packed morning, this is the bowl for you! Coconut
and protein powder supply loads of fiber, healthy fats, and amino acids
for a breakfast that keeps you satisfied until lunch.

SERVES · 1
PREPARATION TIME · 10 MINUTES
COOKING TIME · 5 HOURS

FOR THE OVERNIGHT OAT BASE
1/2 cup rolled oats
1 cup unsweetened almond milk
1 tablespoon chia seeds
2 tablespoons vanilla protein powder
1/4 cup vanilla-flavored coconut yogurt
1/2 tablespoon natural cashew butter

FOR THE TOPPING
1/2 tablespoon natural cashew butter
1 tablespoon crushed cashews
1 teaspoon shredded unsweetened coconut

1 To make the overnight oat base, combine the rolled oats,
almond milk, chia seeds, yogurt, and 1/2 tablespoon cashew
butter in a bowl. Stir to combine, making sure the honey and
cashew butter are incorporated with the other ingredients.

2 Cover the bowl with plastic wrap or a lid and put in the
refrigerator for at least 5 hours, or overnight. As they soak,
the oats and chia will absorb the liquid and attain the consistency
of cooked oatmeal.

3 When the oats are fully soaked, transfer them to a serving
bowl. Top the oat mixture with the 1/2 tablespoon cashew
butter, and finish with the crushed cashews and shredded
coconut. Serve immediately.

Apple Cinnamon Muesli

SERVES · 2
PREPARATION TIME · 7 MINUTES

1 teaspoon cinnamon
2 tablespoons raisins
2 pitted dates, chopped
2 tablespoons buckwheat groats
1/2 cup rolled oats
1/2 cup puffed brown rice cereal
2 tablespoons chopped almonds
2 tablespoons chopped Brazil nuts
2 tablespoons dried apple pieces (chopped dried apple rings)
1/2 large apple, cored and thinly sliced
1 cup unsweetened almond milk
2 teaspoons coconut nectar or pure maple syrup

If you have a busy morning ahead of you, this bowl should be on the menu. Buckwheat groats, oats, and brown rice cereal provide long-lasting energy, while almonds and Brazil nuts add healthy, filling fats. The cinnamon acts as a natural metabolism booster, and the raisins and apple add texture.

1 Combine the cinnamon, raisins, dates, buckwheat groats, oats, rice cereal, almonds, Brazil nuts, and dried apple pieces in a bowl. Mix together, making sure everything is dusted with cinnamon.

2 Divide the muesli between two bowls. Top each bowl with the sliced apple. Pour 1/2 cup of almond milk into each bowl and drizzle each one with 1 teaspoon of coconut nectar or pure maple syrup.

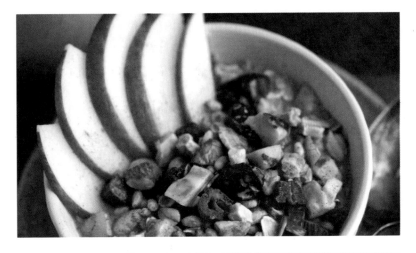

PER SERVING	
Calories	355
Protein	8g
Fat	13g
Carbohydrate	58g
Sugar	24g
Dietary fiber	9g
Vitamins	B
Minerals	iron, magnesium

Try this!
Apricot Coconut Muesli

Apricot and coconut create a wonderful flavor combination, and the nutrients they contain really pack a punch. Dried apricots are rich in vitamin A and contain iron, while coconut is a great source of healthy fats and dietary fiber. Replace the dried apples and dates with 1/4 cup chopped dried apricots and the fresh apple slices with 1/4 cup of toasted coconut flakes, which add even more flavor and texture to the bowl.

Mango Chia Jam & Sweet Cherry

Refreshing, naturally sweet, and full of flavor, this bowl is filling, nutritionally powerful, and surprisingly energizing. Protein- and probiotic-rich Greek yogurt creates a simple base for loads of healthy toppings. The mango chia jam is a great source of vitamin C and fiber, and it combines well with the yogurt, cherries, and banana.

SERVES · 1
PREPARATION TIME · 5 MINUTES
COOKING TIME · 60 MINUTES

FOR THE MANGO CHIA JAM
1 mango, peeled and diced
2 tablespoons unsweetened almond milk
2 teaspoons honey
1 tablespoon chia seeds

FOR THE BOWL
3/4 cup plain Greek yogurt
1/2 medium banana, sliced
1/3 cup pitted sweet cherries
2 tablespoons granola
1 tablespoon pistachios
1 tablespoon unsweetened shredded
   coconut, toasted
2 tablespoons mango chia jam
1/2 teaspoon honey

1 To make the mango chia jam, combine the mango, almond milk, and honey in a blender and process for 1–2 minutes, until semismooth. Transfer the mango mixture to a jar or airtight container, add the chia seeds, and stir to combine. Chill the mixture in the refrigerator for 1 hour, or overnight.

2 When you are ready to serve the breakfast bowl, put the yogurt into a bowl, followed by the banana, cherries, and granola, and sprinkle on the pistachios and coconut. Then top it off with the mango chia jam and honey. Serve immediately.

Try this!
Strawberries & Cream Granola

Swap out the mango for the delicious flavors of strawberries and cream, and gain a boost of antioxidants from the fruit. Make a strawberry chia jam by replacing the mango with 1 cup of fresh strawberries. Omit the cherries from the topping, and drizzle the finished breakfast bowl with 2 tablespoons of canned coconut cream, to add some healthy fats and a delicious creamy coconut finish.

PER SERVING	
Calories	444
Protein	25g
Fat	12g
Carbohydrate	55g
Sugar	41g
Dietary fiber	10g
Vitamins	A, B$_6$, C
Minerals	calcium, potassium

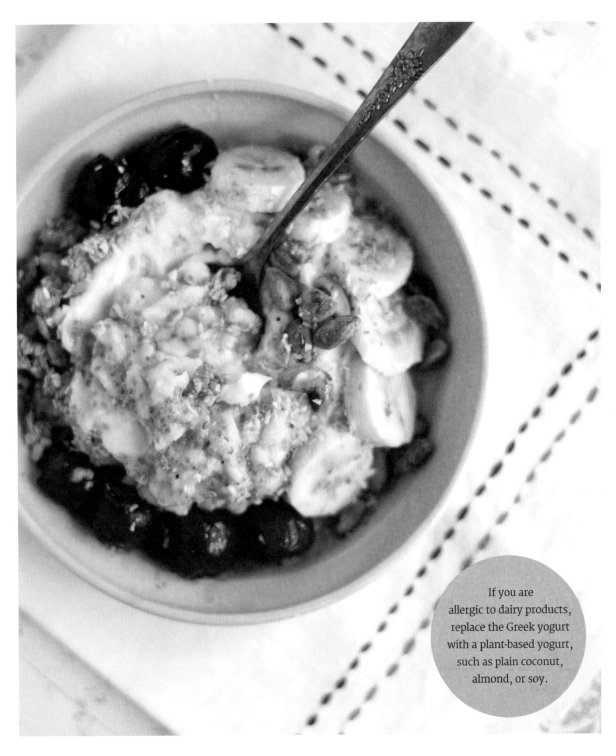

If you are
allergic to dairy products,
replace the Greek yogurt
with a plant-based yogurt,
such as plain coconut,
almond, or soy.

Sweet Potato & Avocado Scramble

SERVES · 2
PREPARATION TIME · 10 MINUTES
COOKING TIME · 40 MINUTES

1 large sweet potato, cut into large cubes
   (about 2 cups)
2 teaspoons olive oil
1 teaspoon salt
1/2 small white onion, diced
1 yellow bell pepper, diced
4 large eggs
4 egg whites
1 teaspoon garlic powder
1/2 teaspoon black pepper
1/2 cup cherry tomatoes, halved
1/2 avocado, diced
1 scallion, chopped
1/2 teaspoon paprika

Sweet potato is loaded with nutrients to get your day started right. It is filling and provides slow-releasing carbohydrates to fuel your body for hours. The flavor blends well with the eggs, avocado, and vegetables. Prepare the sweet potatoes ahead of time and this bowl will be quick to whip up in the morning.

1 Preheat the oven to 400°F. Line a baking pan with parchment paper. Toss the potato cubes with 1 teaspoon olive oil. Distribute them evenly over the baking pan and season with 1/2 teaspoon salt.

2 Roast the potatoes for 15 minutes, then stir them and roast for another 10 minutes, until they are browned all over. Remove from the oven and set aside.

3 Set a nonstick skillet or frying pan over medium heat and add the remaining 1 teaspoon olive oil. When the oil is hot, add the onion and sauté for a few minutes, stirring, until soft and translucent. Add the bell pepper and sauté for 2 minutes, until softened.

4 Add the whole eggs and egg whites and sauté for 5 minutes, mixing them in with the onion and pepper. Stir in the garlic powder and the remaining 1/2 teaspoon of salt, and the pepper.

5 Stir in the tomatoes to heat them through and soften the skins. Add the browned sweet potatoes to the pan and stir to combine. Remove the skillet from the heat and divide the mixture between two bowls.

6 Top the bowls with the diced avocado and chopped scallion, and sprinkle with the paprika. Serve immediately.

PER SERVING	
Calories	439
Protein	25g
Fat	19g
Carbohydrate	40g
Sugar	10g
Dietary fiber	10g
Vitamins	B$_6$, C
Minerals	copper, magnesium

Try this!
Sweet Potato, Bacon & Apple Scramble

Here, the natural sweetness of apples and sweet potato is balanced by the saltiness of beef or nitrate-free pork bacon. Omit the avocado, cherry tomatoes, and bell pepper, and add in strips of chopped, cooked beef or nitrate-free pork bacon with the onion. Add 1 cup of diced apple to the scrambled eggs and sauté for 5 minutes until softened.

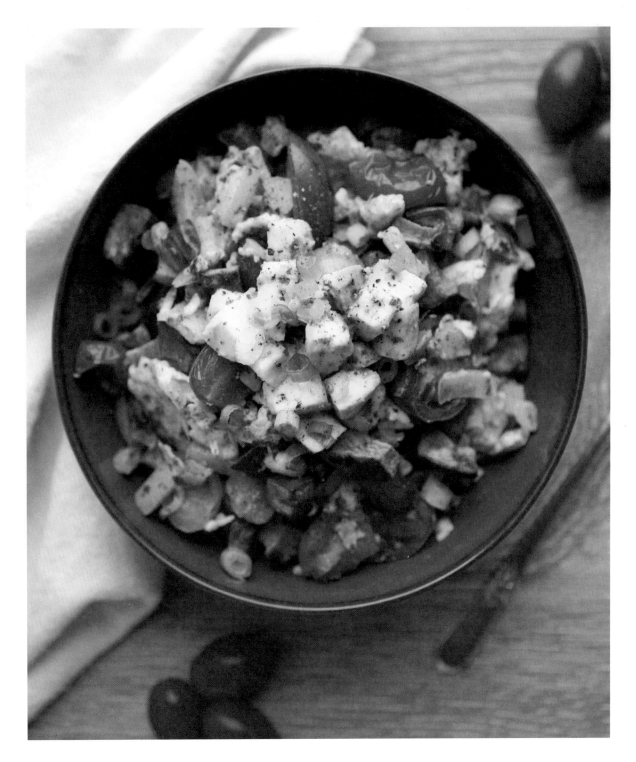

Breakfast Hash

SERVES · 2
PREPARATION TIME · 5 MINUTES
COOKING TIME · 30 MINUTES

1 teaspoon olive oil
1 clove garlic, minced
1/4 cup finely diced onion
1 medium potato, chopped into 1/2-inch
   cubes (1 cup of cubes)
3 organic breakfast sausage links (chicken,
   pork, or beef), removed from their casings
1/2 teaspoon salt
1/2 teaspoon pepper
1/2 teaspoon dried parsley
1/2 teaspoon dried thyme
1 medium red apple, chopped into 1/2-inch
   cubes
1 green bell pepper, diced
1 teaspoon honey
2 large free-range eggs
1 scallion, chopped

This breakfast hash is full of flavor and has a great balance of nutrients to power you all morning. Crispy potatoes supply fiber and vitamins, and taste delicious with the sweet apples. The sausage contains protein to fill you up, and the honey, herbs, bell pepper, and onion add bursts of flavor.

1 Put the olive oil in a large nonstick skillet or frying pan, and set it over medium-high heat. When the oil is hot, add the garlic and onion and sauté for 2–3 minutes, until the onion becomes soft and fragrant.

2 Add the cubed potatoes and sausage meat to the pan. Reduce the heat to medium and sauté for 10 minutes, crumbling the sausage into small pieces with a wooden spoon as it cooks. Season the mixture with the salt, pepper, and dried herbs.

3 Add the apple, bell pepper, and honey to the pan and sauté, stirring occasionally, for 10–12 minutes, until the sausage is browned and the potatoes are cooked through (they should be fork tender).

4 Create two wells in the hash and crack an egg into each well. Cover the skillet with a lid, and cook for 3–4 minutes, or until the eggs are cooked to your preferred doneness.

5 Divide the hash mixture between two bowls and put one egg on top of each one. Sprinkle the chopped scallion evenly over each bowl and serve immediately.

PER SERVING	
Calories	332
Protein	20g
Fat	13g
Carbohydrate	44g
Sugar	16g
Dietary fiber	5g
Vitamins	B_6, C
Minerals	iron

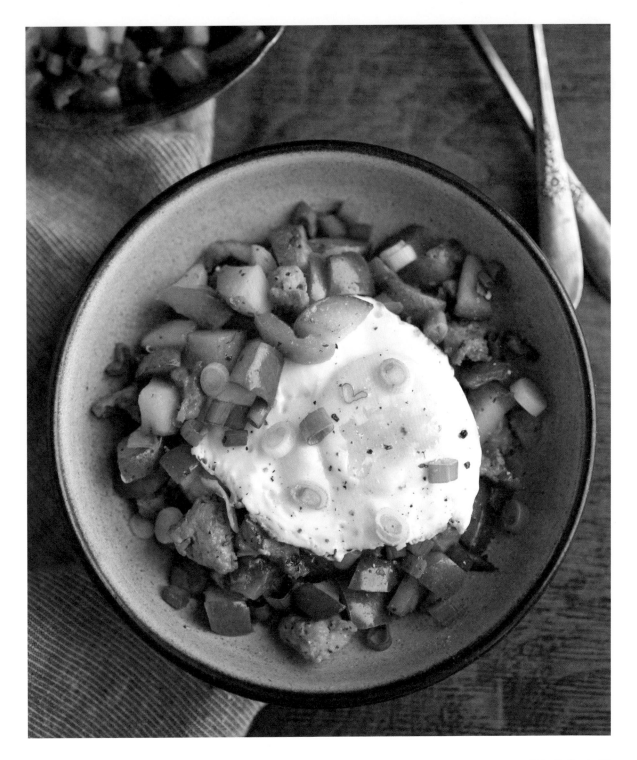

Try this!

Mediterranean Hash

Italian sausage and Greek feta cheese make a great combination. Start the day with a tasty bowl of Mediterranean-inspired flavors that has even more healthy fats than the Breakfast Hash this recipe is based on (see page 74).

SERVES · 2
PREPARATION TIME · 5 MINUTES
COOKING TIME · 30 MINUTES

1 teaspoon olive oil
1 clove garlic, minced
1/4 cup finely diced onion
1 medium potato, chopped into 1/2-inch cubes (1 cup of cubes)
2 Italian sausage links, removed from their casings
1/2 teaspoon salt
1/2 teaspoon pepper
1/2 teaspoon dried parsley
1/2 teaspoon dried thyme
1 cup chopped ripe tomatoes
1/2 cup chopped, pitted Kalamata olives
1 green bell pepper, diced
1 teaspoon honey
2 large free-range eggs
1 tablespoon chopped fresh basil
2 tablespoons crumbled feta

1 Put the olive oil in a large nonstick skillet or frying pan and set it over medium-high heat. When the oil is hot, add the garlic and onion and sauté for 2–3 minutes, until the onion becomes soft and fragrant.

2 Add the cubed potato and sausage meat to the pan. Reduce the heat to medium and sauté for 10 minutes, crumbling the sausage into pieces with a wooden spoon as it cooks. Season the pan with the salt, pepper, and dried herbs.

3 Add the tomatoes, olives, bell pepper, and honey to the pan and sauté, stirring occasionally, for 10–12 minutes, until the sausage is browned and the potato is cooked through (it should be fork tender).

4 Create two wells in the hash and crack an egg into each well. Cover the skillet with a lid, and cook for 3–4 minutes, or until the eggs are cooked to your preferred doneness.

5 Divide the hash mixture between two bowls with one egg on top of each one. Sprinkle chopped basil and crumbled feta evenly over each bowl and serve immediately.

Veggie-loaded Asian Hash

Add some Asian flare to this bowl by combining broccoli and mushrooms with potatoes and sausages. Then intensify the flavors by stirring in soy sauce, sesame oil, and honey.

SERVES · 2
PREPARATION TIME · 5 MINUTES
COOKING TIME · 30 MINUTES

1 teaspoon olive oil
1 clove garlic, minced
1/4 cup finely diced onion
1 medium potato, chopped into 1/2-inch cubes
    (1 cup of cubes)
3 organic breakfast sausage links (chicken,
    pork, or beef), removed from their casings
1/2 teaspoon salt
1/2 teaspoon pepper
1/2 teaspoon dried parsley
1 teaspoon honey
1 tablespoon soy sauce
1 tablespoon sesame oil
1/2 cup finely chopped broccoli florets
1/2 cup sliced mushrooms
1 green bell pepper, diced
2 large free-range eggs
1 scallion, chopped
1 teaspoon toasted sesame seeds

1 Put the olive oil in a large nonstick skillet or frying pan and set it over medium-high heat. When the oil is hot, add the garlic and onion and sauté for 2–3 minutes, until the onion becomes soft and fragrant.

2 Add the cubed potato and sausage meat to the pan. Reduce the heat to medium and sauté for 10 minutes, crumbling the sausage into pieces with a wooden spoon as it cooks. Season the pan with the salt, pepper, and parsley.

3 Combine the honey, soy sauce, and sesame oil in a small bowl and whisk together. Add the mixture to the pan with the broccoli, mushrooms, and bell pepper and sauté, stirring occasionally, for 10–12 minutes, until the sausage is browned and the potato is cooked through (it should be fork tender).

4 Create two wells in the hash and crack an egg into each well. Cover the skillet with a lid, and cook for 3–4 minutes, or until the eggs are cooked to your preferred doneness.

5 Divide the hash mixture between two bowls with one egg on top of each one. Sprinkle the chopped scallion and toasted sesame seeds over each bowl and serve immediately.

Huevos Rancheros

SERVES · 1
PREPARATION TIME · 5 MINUTES
COOKING TIME · 10 MINUTES

1/2 teaspoon olive oil
1/4 cup chopped white onion
1/4 cup canned black beans, drained and
  rinsed
2 tablespoons fresh salsa
1/4 teaspoon salt, plus more if desired
1/4 teaspoon pepper, plus more if desired
2 large free-range eggs
1/2 cup freshly cooked brown rice, kept warm
2 tablespoons prepared guacamole
pinch of dried chipotle peppers
a few sprigs of fresh cilantro
4 tortilla chips
squeeze of fresh lime juice

Wake up to Mexican-inspired flavors. The protein in eggs and black beans keep blood-sugar levels stable and balance the carbohydrates from the rice. Guacamole contains healthy fats, while the salsa, cilantro, and lime burst with flavor. The added crunch of tortilla chips makes this bowl extra good.

1 Set a large skillet or frying pan over medium heat and add the olive oil. When the oil is hot, add the chopped onion and sauté for 2 minutes, until it starts to soften. Add the black beans, 1 tablespoon of the salsa, and the salt and pepper, and continue to sauté for 2 more minutes, until heated through.

2 Create two small wells in the bean mixture and break an egg into each one. Cover the pan with a lid and allow the eggs to cook for 2–3 minutes. Season the eggs with more salt and pepper if desired.

3 Meanwhile, put the warm brown rice in a bowl. As soon as the eggs are cooked to your liking, put the bean mixture on top of the rice and top it with the eggs.

4 Top the mixture with the remaining 1 tablespoon of fresh salsa, the guacamole, dried chipotle, cilantro, and tortilla chips. Squeeze lime juice over the top and serve immediately.

PER SERVING	
Calories	386
Protein	23g
Fat	21g
Carbohydrate	42g
Sugar	4g
Dietary fiber	28g
Vitamins	B₆, C
Minerals	calcium, iron, magnesium

Try this!
Italian Breakfast Eggs

Take your taste buds on a journey from Mexico to Italy. Replace the brown rice with 1/2 cup cooked whole-grain or gluten-free pasta. Omit the black beans, salsa, guacamole, chipotle, cilantro, tortilla chips, and lime juice. Add 1/4 cup tomato basil pasta sauce to the softened onions at the same time as the salt and pepper. When the eggs are cooked, put the cooked pasta in a bowl and top with the tomato mixture and egg. Sprinkle the finished bowl with 1/4 cup chopped fresh basil and 2 tablespoons of shredded mozzarella cheese.

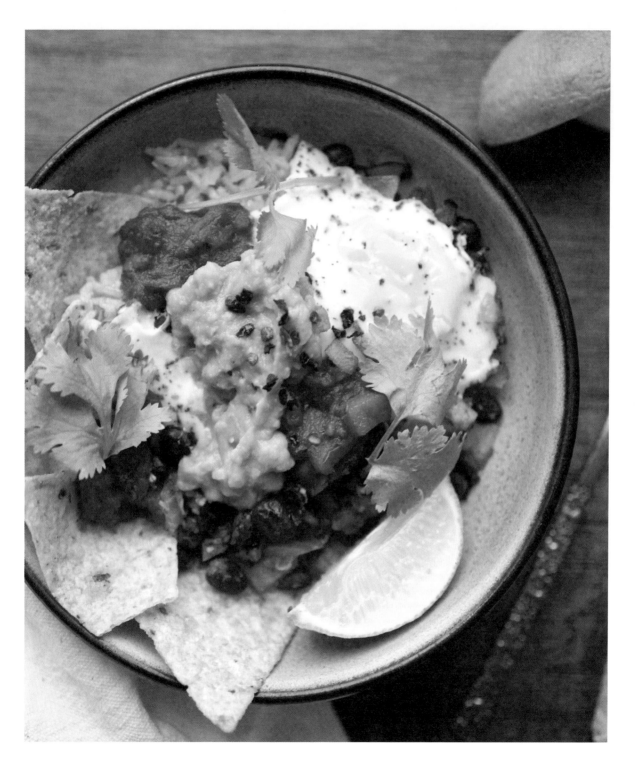

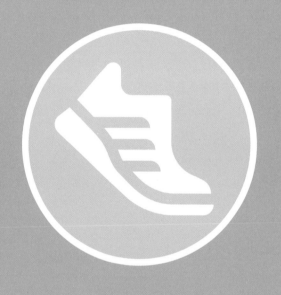

Workout Bowls

When you're working out you need to eat a meal that will supply energy quickly, to support your body during and after exercise. It should contain carbohydrates, proteins, vitamins, and minerals that will help to repair your muscles and satisfy your appetite. You can choose a revitalizing fruit smoothie, a substantial salad, or a warming scramble.

Active Ingredients

Acai Berries
Origin South America
Food Family Palm trees
Nutrients Calcium, carbohydrates, fats, fiber, iron, vitamin A
Power Properties Acai berries are loaded with antioxidants that help promote recovery after exercise by supporting the body to fight inflammation. In this chapter the recipes use a puree of acai berries and other fruits, which can be found in the freezer section of organic or natural grocery stores. Alternatively, you can use acai berry powder.

Edamame Beans
Origin Asia
Food Family Legumes
Nutrients Calcium, carbohydrates, iron, magnesium, protein, vitamins B6 and C
Power Properties Edamame beans are a variety of soy bean. They are rich in performance-boosting protein—17g per cup—and are a fantastic source of amino acids for those who follow a plant-based diet. Choose organic, non-GMO, frozen, shelled beans. Steam, or let them thaw, before eating.

Greek Yogurt and Alternatives
Origin Greece
Food Family Dairy
Nutrients Calcium, probiotics, protein, vitamin B12
Power Properties Greek yogurt has as much as 18g of protein per serving. It is also high in probiotics that promote intestinal health and digestive function. Always use plain, unsweetened yogurt to avoid added sugars or artificial ingredients. If you are unable to eat cow's dairy products, use a plant-based yogurt, such as plain coconut or soy. If you eat a nondairy yogurt before or after a workout, consider adding protein powder to increase the protein content.

Matcha

Origin Asia
Food Family Theaceae
Nutrients Chromium, manganese, selenium, zinc
Power Properties Matcha is a powder made from green tea leaves. It is ideal before or after a workout, as it provides energy along with antioxidants to boost recovery. Green tea contains epigallocatechin-3-gallate, an antioxidant more powerful than vitamin C or E.

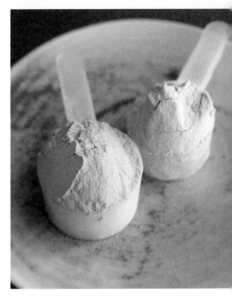

Protein powder

Protein Powder

Origin First produced in the United States and Europe
Food Family N/A
Nutrients Protein/amino acids, and added vitamins and minerals
Power Properties Muscles work hard during workouts and need support to give the body additional power and stamina. Protein powder is a source of amino acids and is available in several varieties. Choose an organic, natural grass-fed whey or plant-based protein powder that has a blend of two or more of the following ingredients: hemp, brown rice, pea, or soy. Make sure there are no artificial ingredients, additives, or refined sweeteners. For the recipes requiring vanilla, chocolate, and hemp-based protein powders, look for ones that are naturally flavored.

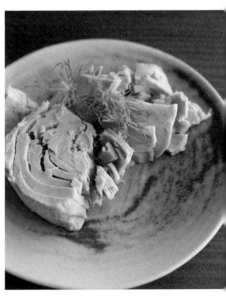

Tuna

Tuna

Origin Various
Food Family Scombridae
Nutrients Omega-3 fatty acids, phosphorus, protein, selenium, vitamins B3, B6, B12, and D
Power Properties This saltwater fish holds all the essential amino acids that help to promote muscle growth, strength, and repair. Tuna also has vitamin D, which is important for athletic performance, as it has a direct impact on the health of skeletal muscle tissue and is needed for energy. Make sure to buy sustainably sourced fish.

Tropical Smoothie

SERVES · 1
PREPARATION TIME · 7 MINUTES

FOR THE BASE
1/2 cup frozen banana chunks
1/2 cup frozen pineapple chunks
1/2 cup mango chunks
1 cup unsweetened vanilla almond milk
1 heaping tablespoon ground flaxseed
1 scoop vanilla protein powder

FOR THE TOPPING
1 tablespoon toasted shredded unsweetened
   coconut
1 teaspoon chia seeds
1 tablespoon granola
1 tablespoon sliced pineapple
a few slices of banana

Transport yourself to the beach with this tropical-inspired smoothie. It combines quickly absorbed protein powder, to promote muscle-building and repair, with vitamins and antioxidants from the banana, pineapple, and mango. Enjoy this bowl 1 hour before exercise.

1 Combine the frozen banana, frozen pineapple, mango, almond milk, flaxseed, and protein powder in a blender and process for 1–2 minutes, until thick and smooth. Transfer to a bowl.

2 Top the bowl with the toasted coconut, chia seeds, granola, and sliced fresh pineapple and banana.

PER SERVING	
Calories	429
Protein	31g
Fat	12g
Carbohydrate	42g
Sugar	27g
Dietary fiber	11g
Vitamins	A, C
Minerals	calcium, iron

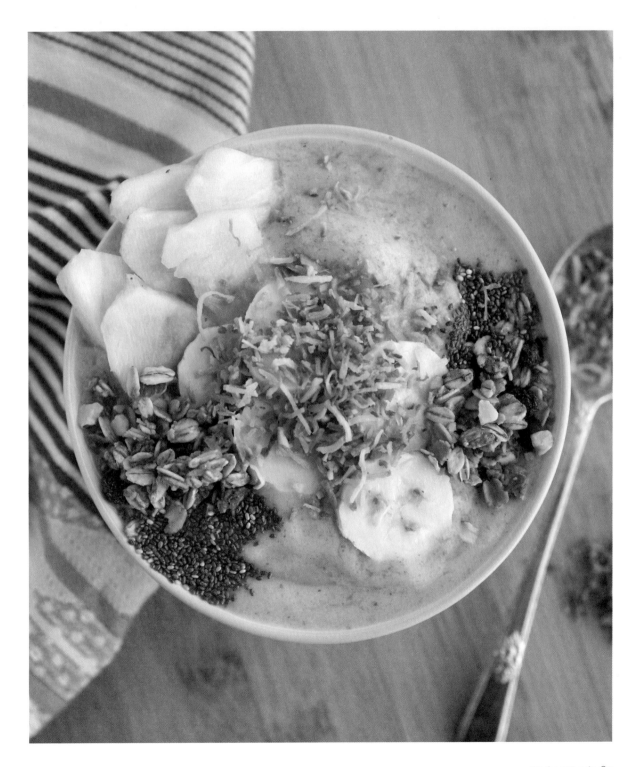

Try this!

Kiwi & Pineapple Smoothie

Add delicious kiwifruit to this tropical mix to bring in a major boost of vitamin C. This variation of the recipe on page 84 also replaces the mango with an extra helping of refreshing pineapple.

SERVES · 1
PREPARATION TIME · 7 MINUTES

1/2 cup frozen banana chunks
1 cup frozen pineapple chunks
1 cup unsweetened vanilla almond milk
1 heaping tablespoon ground flaxseed
1 scoop vanilla protein powder
1 tablespoon toasted shredded unsweetened coconut
1 teaspoon chia seeds
1 tablespoon granola of choice
1 kiwifruit, sliced

1 Combine the frozen banana, frozen pineapple, almond milk, flaxseed, and protein powder in a blender and process for 1–2 minutes, until thick and smooth. Transfer to a bowl.

2 Top the bowl with the toasted coconut, chia seeds, granola, and sliced kiwifruit.

Mango & Chili Smoothie

Turn up the heat with this spicy and refreshing recipe.
Researchers have found that capsacin—the compound
in red pepper flakes that gives them their heat—may stimulate
the body to burn energy, create heat, and boost metabolism.

SERVES · 1
PREPARATION TIME · 7 MINUTES

1/2 cup frozen banana chunks
1 cup mango chunks
1 cup unsweetened vanilla almond milk
1 heaping tablespoon ground flaxseed
1 scoop vanilla protein powder
1/2 teaspoon red pepper flakes, plus extra
   to sprinkle
1 tablespoon toasted shredded
   unsweetened coconut
1 teaspoon chia seeds
1 tablespoon granola
2 tablespoons sliced fresh mango

1 Combine the frozen banana, mango, almond milk, flaxseed, protein powder, and red pepper flakes in a blender and process for 1–2 minutes, until thick and smooth. Transfer to a bowl.

2 Top the bowl with the toasted coconut, chia seeds, granola, and sliced fresh mango, then sprinkle with red pepper flakes.

Goji Berry, Hemp & Acai

SERVES · 4
PREPARATION TIME · 10 MINUTES

FOR THE BASE
1 (3½ ounce) package acai berry puree or
   2 heaping tablespoons acai berry powder
2 cups frozen mixed berries
2 frozen bananas, peeled and diced
2 cups unsweetened almond milk

FOR THE TOPPING
½ cup shredded coconut
1 fresh banana, peeled and sliced
¼ cup dried goji berries
¼ cup hempseeds
4 teaspoons honey
½ cup granola

Acai berries are loaded with antioxidants and provide ample amounts of preworkout fuel. Top the base of this bowl with chewy goji berries, which are rich in vitamin A, selenium, and iron, and hempseeds, which are loaded with protein. Enjoy one of these bowls 30–60 minutes before exercise.

1 Combine the acai berry puree or powder, mixed berries, frozen bananas, and almond milk in a blender and process for 1–2 minutes, until thick and smooth.

2 Divide the acai mixture evenly among four bowls.

3 Top the bowls with the shredded coconut, sliced banana, goji berries, hempseeds, honey, and granola. Serve immediately.

PER SERVING	
Calories	412
Protein	9g
Fat	18g
Carbohydrate	50g
Sugar	33g
Dietary fiber	9g
Vitamins	A
Minerals	iron, selenium

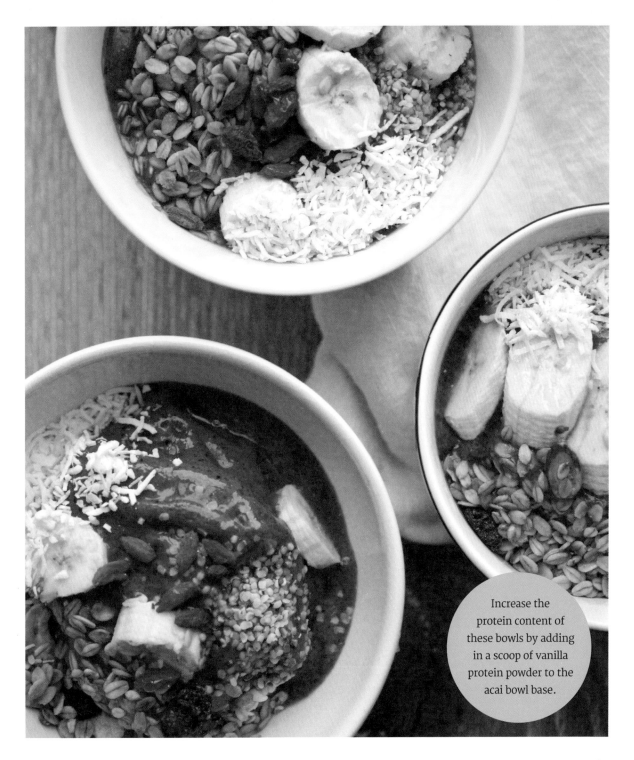

Increase the protein content of these bowls by adding in a scoop of vanilla protein powder to the acai bowl base.

Try this!

Matcha & Acai

Increase the amount of iron and vitamins A and C in this acai bowl by adding raw spinach leaves, and improve the energy-boosting benefits with matcha green tea powder.

SERVES · 4
PREPARATION TIME · 10 MINUTES

FOR THE BASE
2 cups raw spinach
1 (3½ ounce) package acai berry puree or
   2 heaping tablespoons acai berry powder
2 cups frozen mixed berries
2 frozen bananas, peeled and diced
2 cups unsweetened almond milk
4 teaspoons matcha powder

FOR THE TOPPING
½ cup shredded coconut
1 fresh banana, peeled and sliced
4 teaspoons honey
½ cup granola

1 Combine the spinach, acai berry puree or powder, mixed berries, frozen bananas, almond milk, and matcha in a blender and process for 1–2 minutes, until thick and smooth.

2 Divide the acai mixture evenly among four bowls.

3 Top the bowls with the shredded coconut, sliced banana, honey, and granola. Serve immediately.

Try this!

Chocolate Protein & Acai

When you're exercising, your body benefits from antioxidants,
which help build and repair muscles. Add the nutrients you need
by including protein powder and cocoa nibs in the acai bowl.

SERVES · 4
PREPARATION TIME · 10 MINUTES

FOR THE BASE
2 scoops chocolate protein powder
1 (3½ ounce) package acai berry puree or
   2 heaping tablespoons acai berry powder
2 cups frozen mixed berries
2 frozen bananas, peeled and diced
2½ cups unsweetened almond milk

FOR THE TOPPING
½ cup shredded coconut
1 fresh banana, peeled and sliced
¼ cup cocoa nibs
4 teaspoons honey
½ cup granola

1 Combine the chocolate protein powder, acai berry puree or
powder, mixed berries, frozen bananas, and almond milk in
a blender and process for 1–2 minutes, until thick and smooth.

2 Divide the acai mixture evenly among four bowls.

3 Top the bowls with the shredded coconut, sliced banana,
cocoa nibs, honey, and granola. Serve immediately.

Chocolate, Hazelnut & Hemp

SERVES · 1
PREPARATION TIME · 5 MINUTES

FOR THE BASE
1 medium banana, peeled, cut into chunks, and frozen
1/2 cup frozen strawberries
5 ice cubes
3/4 cup hazelnut milk (or unsweetened almond milk)
1/4 cup chocolate hemp protein powder
1 heaping tablespoon cocoa powder (or raw cocoa powder)

FOR THE TOPPING
1–2 strawberries, sliced
1 teaspoon cocoa nibs
1 teaspoon hempseeds
1 teaspoon 70% dark chocolate shavings
1 teaspoon chopped raw hazelnuts

It's hard to believe that this is a workout bowl and not a dreamy dessert—it could certainly pass for one. The hazelnuts supply iron, vitamin B6, and magnesium, and complement the chocolate and cocoa, which add calcium, too. Enjoy this bowl 1 hour before exercise, or 15–45 minutes afterward.

1 Combine the frozen banana and strawberries, ice cubes, hazelnut milk, protein powder, and cocoa powder in a blender and process for 1–2 minutes, until thick and smooth.

2 Pour the mixture into a bowl. Top with the sliced strawberries, cocoa nibs, hempseeds, chocolate shavings, and chopped hazelnuts. Serve immediately.

Try this!
Vanilla, Chai & Hazelnut

Combine the hazelnuts with vanilla and chai spice mix for a lighter flavor. Replace the cocoa powder with 1 teaspoon of chai tea powder and the chocolate hemp protein powder with a vanilla hemp protein powder. Omit the cocoa nibs and chocolate shavings from the bowl toppings and replace them with 1/4 teaspoon of ground cinnamon.

PER SERVING	
Calories	404
Protein	26g
Fat	14g
Carbohydrate	63g
Sugar	29g
Dietary fiber	18g
Vitamins	B$_6$
Minerals	calcium, iron, magnesium

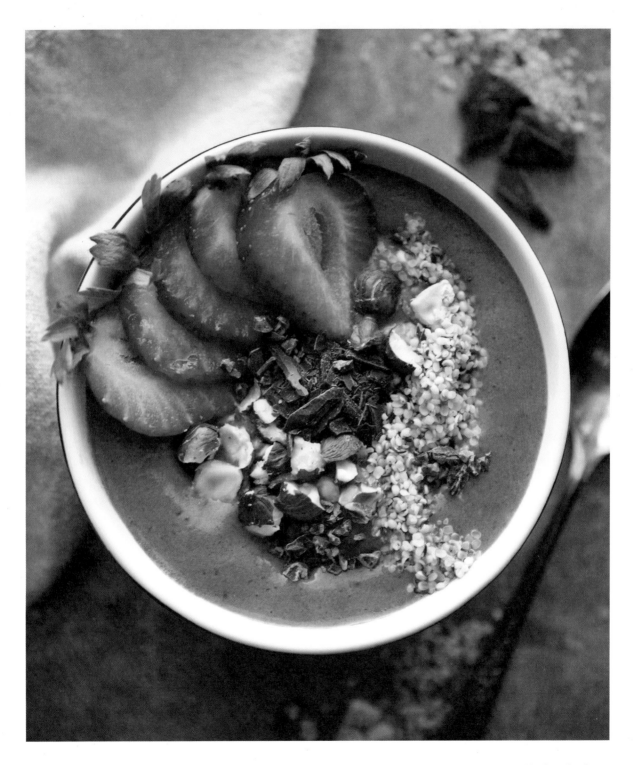

Peanut Butter, Banana & Blueberry Pancakes

SERVES · 2
PREPARATION TIME · 5 MINUTES
COOKING TIME · 10 MINUTES

2 ripe medium bananas, peeled
1 tablespoon almond flour
1 whole egg
2 egg whites
2 tablespoons peanut butter
1/4 teaspoon baking powder
1/2 teaspoon pure vanilla extract
1/8 teaspoon salt
1/3 cup plus 2 tablespoons fresh blueberries
1 tablespoon pure maple syrup

Pancakes are always a good idea—especially when combined with peanut butter, maple syrup, and blueberries. Here, eggs and almond flour deliver protein, while bananas add carbohydrates that are quick to digest. Enjoy these pancakes 30–60 minutes before exercise or 30–60 minutes afterward.

1 To make the pancake batter, combine the bananas, almond flour, egg, egg whites, 1 tablespoon peanut butter, baking powder, vanilla extract, and salt in a blender. Process on low speed for 20–30 seconds until well incorporated and mostly smooth, but with some small chunks of banana remaining. Transfer the batter to a bowl and stir in 1/3 cup fresh blueberries.

2 Heat a griddle or a large nonstick skillet over medium heat and grease lightly with coconut oil or cooking spray. Pour "sand dollar" sized portions (about 3 inches in diameter) of the batter onto the pan or griddle and cook for 2–3 minutes on one side. When the pancakes begin to lightly bubble, turn them over and cook for 1–2 minutes on the other side, until lightly browned. Stack the cooked pancakes on a plate to keep them warm. Repeat until you have made ten pancakes.

3 Create two stacks of five pancakes and cut them evenly into quarters. Divide the quartered pancakes between two bowls and top with the remaining fresh blueberries, then drizzle with peanut butter and pure maple syrup. Serve immediately.

PER SERVING	
Calories	386
Protein	23g
Fat	21g
Carbohydrate	42g
Sugar	23g
Dietary fiber	28g
Vitamins	B₆, C
Minerals	calcium, iron, magnesium

Try this!
Orange, Chocolate & Coconut Pancakes

Increase the protein and add a dose of antioxidants by replacing the almond flour with 2 tablespoons of chocolate protein powder. Omit the peanut butter and add 1 tablespoon of fresh orange juice to the batter. Replace the blueberries with 1/4 cup plus 2 tablespoons dark chocolate chips. Replace the peanut butter in the topping with 1 tablespoon dark chocolate chips, 1 tablespoon toasted coconut flakes, and 1/2 teaspoon fresh orange zest for each bowl. Finish with the pure maple syrup.

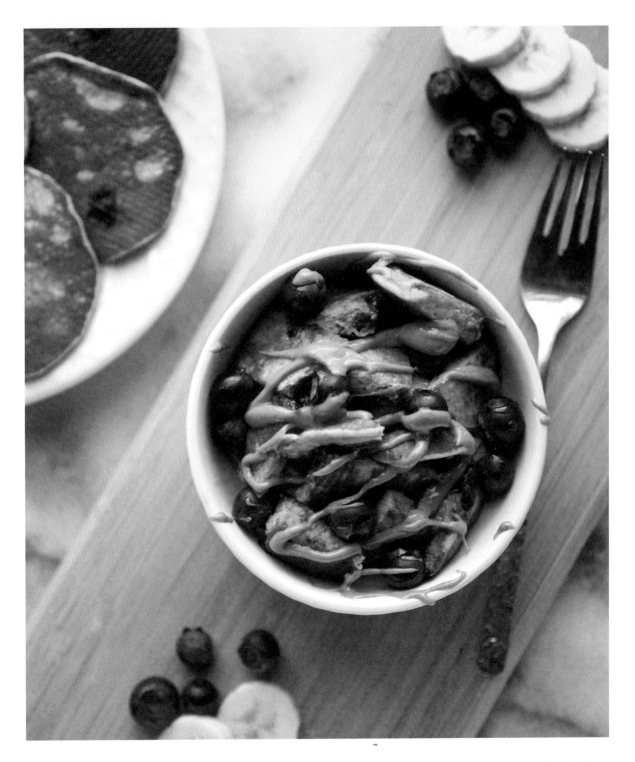

Try this!

Peanut Butter, Cherry & Macadamia Pancakes

Cherries contain potassium, which can prevent postexercise pain caused by inflammation. Plus they taste delicious when combined with protein-packed macadamia nuts and hempseeds.

SERVES · 2
PREPARATION TIME · 5 MINUTES
COOKING TIME · 10 MINUTES

2 ripe medium bananas, peeled
1 tablespoon almond flour
1 whole egg
2 egg whites
1 tablespoon peanut butter
1/4 teaspoon baking powder
1/2 teaspoon pure vanilla extract
1/8 teaspoon salt
1/2 cup plus 1 tablespoon pitted and chopped fresh cherries
3 tablespoons chopped macadamia nuts
1 tablespoon pure maple syrup

1 To make the pancake batter, combine the bananas, almond flour, egg, egg whites, peanut butter, baking powder, vanilla extract, and salt in a blender. Process on low speed for 20–30 seconds, until well incorporated and mostly smooth, but with some small chunks of banana remaining.

2 Transfer the batter to a bowl and stir in 1/4 cup pitted and chopped fresh cherries and 2 tablespoons of chopped macadamia nuts.

3 Cook as for the Peanut Butter, Banana & Blueberry Pancakes on page 94.

4 Create two stacks of five pancakes and cut them evenly into quarters. Divide the quartered pancakes between two bowls and top with 1 tablespoon of pitted and chopped cherries and 1 tablespoon of chopped macadamia nuts.

5 Combine the remaining 1/4 cup of pitted chopped cherries and the maple syrup in a small saucepan and cook over low heat until heated through, mashing the cherries lightly with a fork to let out the juices and create a chunky maple cherry syrup. Divide this syrup between the two bowls, drizzling the syrup over the pancake pieces. Serve immediately.

Berry Green Smoothie

With its rich, deep purple hue, you probably wouldn't guess that this bowl is loaded with healthy greens! Frozen berries provide antioxidants and carbohydrates, while the spinach is rich in iron. Enjoy 15–30 minutes after a workout. Depending on the protein powder you use, this recipe can be vegan or dairy-free.

SERVES · 1
PREPARATION TIME · 5 MINUTES

1/2 cup fresh or frozen spinach leaves
1/2 teaspoons matcha green tea powder
1/2 cup frozen blackberries
1/2 cup frozen raspberries
1/2 cup natural orange juice
1 scoop natural or vanilla protein powder of
    choice
2 tablespoons granola
2–3 sprigs of mint
1 teaspoon crushed pistachios

1 Combine the spinach, matcha, frozen berries, orange juice, and protein powder in a blender and process for 1–2 minutes, until smooth and thick.

2 Transfer the berry mixture to a bowl and top with the granola, mint, and pistachios. Serve immediately.

PER SERVING	
Calories	341
Protein	31g
Fat	4g
Carbohydrate	39g
Sugar	23g
Dietary fiber	14g
Vitamins	A, B_6, C
Minerals	calcium, iron, magnesium

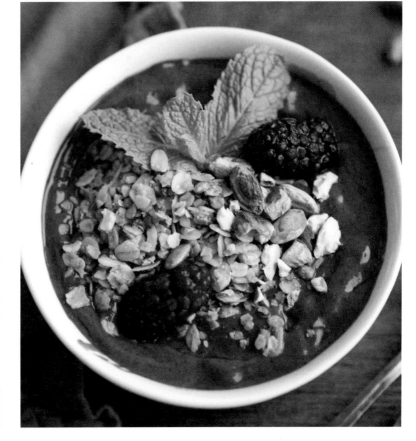

Apple, Pecan & Caramel Crunch

SERVES · 1
PREPARATION TIME · 5 MINUTES
COOKING TIME · 5 MINUTES

FOR THE CARAMEL SAUCE
1/4 teaspoon tapioca flour
2 tablespoons full-fat canned coconut milk
1 tablespoon pure maple syrup
1/4 teaspoon pure vanilla extract
pinch sea salt

FOR THE BOWL
3/4 cup plain Greek yogurt
1/2 medium apple, diced
2 tablespoons bran, spelt, or rice flakes
2 tablespoons buckwheat groats
1 tablespoon chopped pecans
1 tablespoon caramel sauce

Apple, pecans, and caramel top the protein-rich Greek yogurt in this tasty bowl. Added crunch comes from the grain flakes and buckwheat groats, which deliver long-lasting energy. The coconut milk contains healthy fats. Enjoy this bowl 60–90 minutes before a workout or longer endurance exercise.

1 To make the caramel sauce, combine the tapioca flour and coconut milk in a bowl and whisk until smooth. Heat a small saucepan over medium heat and add the coconut milk mixture, maple syrup, vanilla extract, and salt. Whisk continuously until smooth and bubbling. Simmer for 2–3 minutes, until reduced and slightly thickened, then remove from the heat and set aside.

2 Spoon the yogurt into a bowl and top with the diced apple, bran, spelt or rice flakes, buckwheat, and chopped pecans. Drizzle with 1 tablespoon of the caramel sauce and serve immediately. The remaining caramel sauce can be stored in a screw top jar in the refrigerator for up to 3 days.

Try this!
Fig, Pistachio & Caramel Yogurt

Replace the apples with fiber- and vitamin-rich fresh figs and antioxidant-rich pistachios. Figs and pistachios also make a fantastic flavor combination when combined with the sweet caramel sauce and velvety protein-packed yogurt. Simply swap out the diced apples for 2 fresh figs, quartered, and replace the pecans with 1 tablespoon of chopped pistachios. Keep the flakes and buckwheat, for their healthy complex carbohydrates, and drizzle over the caramel sauce.

PER SERVING	
Calories	329
Protein	22g
Fat	9g
Carbohydrate	44g
Sugar	23g
Dietary fiber	6g
Vitamins	C
Minerals	calcium, iron

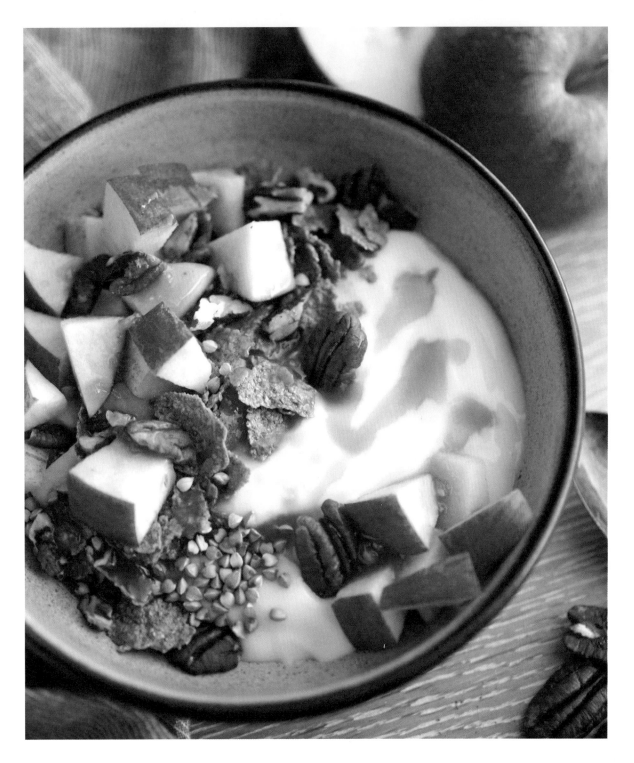

Greek Chicken & Chickpea

SERVES · 2
PREPARATION TIME · 5 MINUTES
COOKING TIME · 15 MINUTES

FOR THE DRESSING
1 tablespoon red wine vinegar
1/2 tablespoon olive oil
2 tablespoons fresh lemon juice
pinch of oregano
salt and pepper

FOR THE SALAD
1/2 cup diced cucumber
1/2 cup diced tomato
1/2 cup diced red bell pepper
1/4 cup diced red onion
1/2 cup cooked and shredded rotisserie
   chicken breast
1/4 cup diced olives
1/2 cup cooked chickpeas
2 tablespoons crumbled goat, sheep,
   or cow's milk feta

If you are craving something savory before or after your workout, this bowl is just what you need. It is loaded with fresh, nutrient-rich vegetables, and chicken, which is rich in amino acids that help build and repair muscles. Enjoy this dish 30 minutes before a workout, or 15–30 minutes afterward.

1 Combine the red wine vinegar, olive oil, lemon juice, and oregano in a small bowl and season with salt and pepper. Whisk the ingredients together and set them aside.

2 Combine the cucumber, tomato, bell pepper, onion, chicken, olives, chickpeas, and cheese in a larger bowl.

3 Pour over the dressing and mix well to combine. Let the salad chill for at least 15 minutes, or up to several hours, in the refrigerator (the longer the better as the flavors intensify) and then divide it evenly between two bowls and serve immediately.

Try this!
Greek Vegan Edamame

If you aren't a meat or dairy eater, try a healthy and protein-packed vegan version of this recipe. Simply swap out the shredded chicken breast for 1/2 cup shelled edamame beans. Edamame beans contain ample amounts of plant-based protein, as well as dietary fiber, iron, magnesium, and manganese, which are all beneficial to performance. Replace the feta cheese with another healthy fat—avocado. Add 2 tablespoons of diced avocado to the salad instead.

PER SERVING	
Calories	196
Protein	15g
Fat	7g
Carbohydrate	14g
Sugar	4g
Dietary fiber	3g
Vitamins	A, B_6, C
Minerals	iron, magnesium

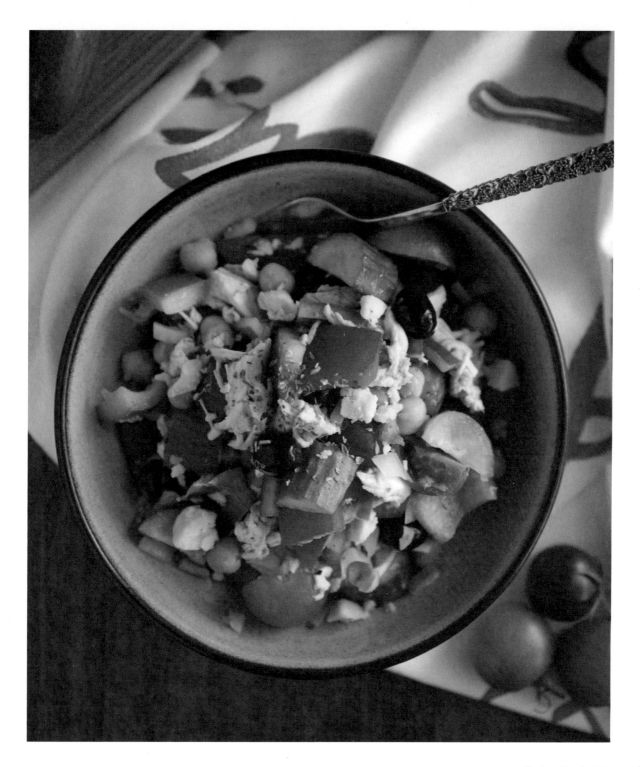

Creamy Tuna Pasta Salad

SERVES · 2
PREPARATION TIME · 5 MINUTES

FOR THE DRESSING
1 tablespoon finely chopped shallot
1 tablespoon chopped fresh basil
1 tablespoon plus 1 teaspoon olive oil
1 tablespoon apple cider vinegar
1 tablespoon lemon juice
1 teaspoon honey
salt and freshly ground black pepper

FOR THE BOWLS
1¼ cups whole wheat or gluten-free pasta of
   choice, cooked and cooled
1 (4-ounce) can (drained weight) tuna
2 teaspoons chopped capers
6 sun-dried tomatoes, chopped
⅓ cup garden peas
½ cup chopped cherry tomatoes
1 teaspoon lemon zest
chopped fresh parsley

This bowl contains the Mediterranean flavors of basil, lemon, sun-dried tomatoes, and capers. Tuna is a great source of protein and, when combined with whole wheat pasta, it provides fuel for an endurance workout. This dish is perfect 60-minutes preworkout or 30–60 minutes postworkout.

1 Cook the pasta following the instructions on the package and let it cool. Combine the shallot, basil, olive oil, cider vinegar, lemon juice, honey, salt, and freshly ground black pepper in a small food processor, or single-serve blender, and blend until emulsified. Set the dressing aside. Alternatively, combine the dressing ingredients in a jar and shake vigorously until emulsified.

2 Combine the cooked and cooled pasta, tuna, capers, sun-dried tomatoes, peas, cherry tomatoes, lemon zest, and chopped parsley in a large bowl and mix well to combine.

3 Pour in the dressing and mix again until everything is well coated. Serve immediately, or store in the refrigerator for a few hours to let the flavors intensify.

PER SERVING	
Calories	304
Protein	20g
Fat	11g
Carbohydrate	36g
Sugar	7g
Dietary fiber	3g
Vitamins	A, B, C
Minerals	calcium, iron, magnesium

Try this!
Creamy Tuna Bow Tie Pasta Salad

Try a delicious, creamy dressing in this simple variation with a mayonnaise dressing. Add crunch and more textures by bringing in vitamin C-rich broccoli and calcium-rich Cheddar cheese. This will fuel your body before a longer endurance workout. Consume about 2 hours before exercise. Use bow tie pasta (gluten-free if desired) for the bowls, and swap out the sun-dried tomatoes and capers for ½ cup of chopped broccoli florets. Omit the lemon zest and add ¼ cup of cubed Cheddar cheese (or use a dairy-free cheese if desired).

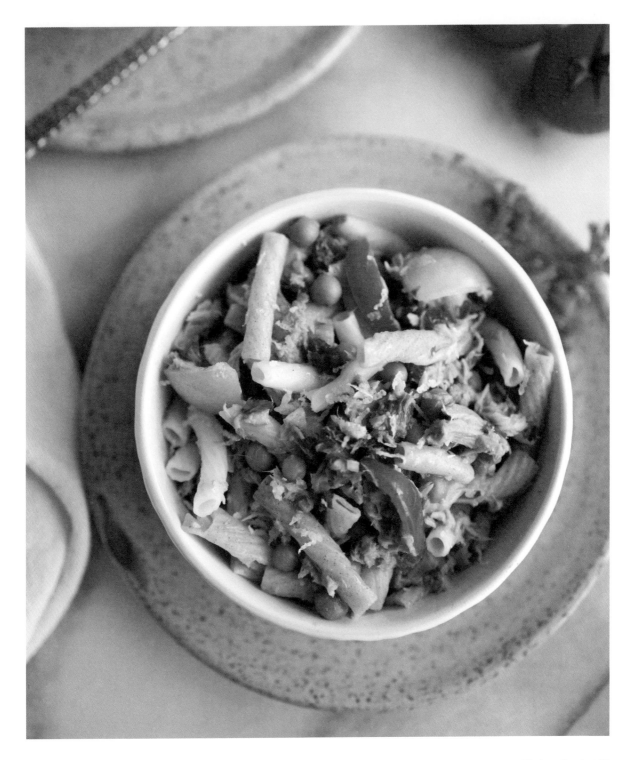

Salmon, Lemon & Quinoa Scramble

SERVES · 1
PREPARATION TIME · 10 MINUTES
COOKING TIME · 5 MINUTES

FOR THE DRESSING
1/2 tablespoon mayonnaise
1 tablespoon lemon juice
1 tablespoon chopped fresh dill
1/8 teaspoon garlic powder
1/2 teaspoon honey
pinch of salt and pepper

FOR THE BOWL
1 whole egg and 2 large egg whites
pinch of salt and pepper
11/2 ounces chopped smoked salmon
1/2 cup cooked quinoa
1 teaspoon chopped red onion
1 teaspoon capers
sprigs of fresh dill

Protein-packed salmon contains omega-rich fats, as well as vitamins B_6 and B_{12}. Here it is combined with quinoa for sustained energy and a creamy-yet-light lemon dressing that adds antioxidants and flavor. Enjoy this dish 60–90 minutes before a workout or 30–60 minutes postworkout.

1 Combine the mayonnaise, lemon juice, dill, garlic powder, honey, and a pinch of salt and pepper in a small bowl, and whisk until smooth. Set it aside.

2 Combine the egg and egg whites in another bowl, season with salt and pepper, and whisk to combine.

3 Heat a medium-sized saucepan over medium heat, and, once hot, add the whisked eggs and scramble for 1–2 minutes. Add the smoked salmon and scramble for another 1–2 minutes, until the eggs are cooked through.

4 Add the cooked quinoa to the pan and sauté with the eggs and salmon for 1 more minute to heat it through. Transfer the mixture to a bowl and drizzle with the dressing and garnish with the chopped red onion, capers, and dill. Serve immediately.

PER SERVING	
Calories	331
Protein	26g
Fat	14g
Carbohydrate	24g
Sugar	1g
Dietary fiber	3g
Vitamins	B_6, B_{12}
Minerals	calcium, iron, magnesium

Try this!
Santa Fe Salmon Scramble

Add a taste of Santa Fe to this delicious combination of scrambled eggs and smoked salmon. Black beans boost athletic performance 1 hour preworkout, and corn provides magnesium, iron, and vitamin B6. Swap out the cooked quinoa for 1/2 cup of black beans (canned, drained, and rinsed). Omit all of the dressing ingredients. Prepare the scramble and add 1 tablespoon of salsa with the salmon. When the eggs are cooked, add the beans and corn. Transfer the scramble to a bowl, and top with 1 tablespoon of chopped chives.

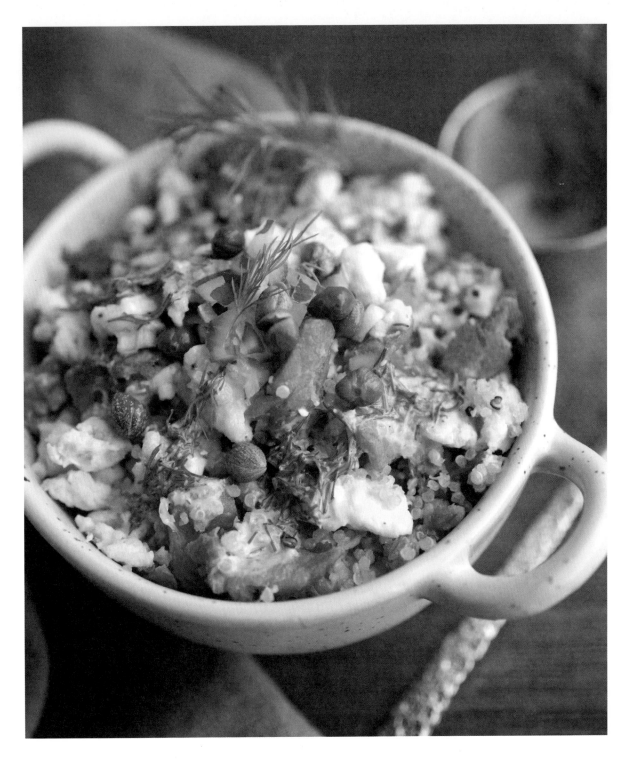

Small Bowls

When choosing what to eat between meals, it's important to look for snacks that are filling, give you energy, vitamins, and minerals, and help balance your blood sugar. Salad bowls are a great way to do this, whether you enjoy them at home, made fresh with warm ingredients, or in your lunch bag at work.

Active Ingredients

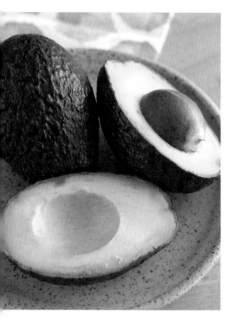

Avocados

Avocados

Origin South Central Mexico

Food Family Lauraceae

Nutrients Copper, fiber, folate, omega essential fatty acids, potassium, vitamins B5, B6, C, E, and K

Power Properties Avocados contain unsaturated fats that are rich in Omega-3, which is essential for brain and nervous system health. They have been linked to improved memory, mood, and cognitive function. To check if an avocado is ripe, remove the stem and look underneath: If it is green it is ripe, yellow means it is not ripe, and brown means it is overripe.

Hummus

Origin Middle East

Food Family Various

Nutrients Fiber, carbohydrates, copper, folate, iron, manganese, magnesium, phosphorus, protein, vitamins B1, B6

Power Properties This traditional dish is made from chickpeas, blended with tahini, olive oil, garlic, lemon juice, and spices. The chickpeas add slow-releasing carbohydrates and fiber, and the fats from the oil add omega-rich fatty acids. If you buy hummus from a store, look for one without artificial ingredients.

Rice Vermicelli Noodles

Origin Asia

Food Family Grasses

Nutrients Carbohydrates, fiber, manganese, protein, selenium

Power Properties These very thin noodles can be made with white or brown rice, or a combination of both. They are a quick way to add fast-digesting carbohydrates to a meal. For longer lasting energy, brown or a combination of brown and white rice noodles are best. Look for packages with rice, as the only ingredient, or tapioca flour as the only addition.

Tahini (or Sesame Paste)

Origin Middle East

Food Family Pedaliaceae

Nutrients Copper, calcium, fat, fiber, iron, magnesium, manganese, phosphorus, zinc

Power Properties This paste made from ground sesame seeds has a subtle, nutty taste. It makes a creamy addition to power bowls, adding bone-building minerals, filling fiber, polyunsaturated fats, and phytosterols, which have been linked to healthy cholesterol levels. It adds a dairy-free richness to salad dressings. Look for brands that contain only sesame seeds, or sesame seeds and olive oil.

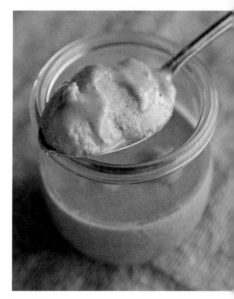

Tahini

Tofu, Extra Firm

Origin China

Food Family Legume

Nutrients Calcium, copper, manganese, omega essential fatty acids, phosphorus, protein, selenium

Power Properties Tofu is a plant-based protein made from soy milk. It has been linked to improved cardiovascular health. It has a mild flavor, so it works best when marinated or combined with a flavorful sauce. The firmer the tofu, the higher the protein content. Because tofu is made from soybeans, buying non-GMO organic tofu is best.

Zucchini (Summer Squash)

Origin Italy

Food Family Cucurbits

Nutrients Copper, fiber, magnesium, manganese, phosphorus, potassium, vitamin C

Power Properties Zucchini is a versatile vegetable that can be enjoyed raw, steamed, roasted, sautéed, or even baked in breads and muffins. It has plenty of antioxidants and fiber. Studies have found that zucchini aids the metabolism of sugar, which in turn regulates blood-sugar levels.

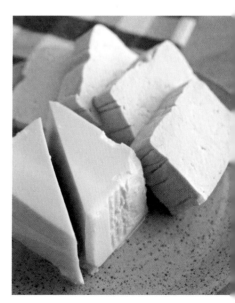

Tofu

Vitality Superfood Salad

This bowl may be small, but it packs in plenty of nutrients. It is loaded with vitamin-rich vegetables, detoxifying herbs, protein-packed chicken, and antioxidant-rich blueberries. They help to improve skin, hair, and nail health, and benefit joints, bones, and the cardiovascular system.

SERVES · 2
PREPARATION TIME · 10 MINUTES

FOR THE BOWL
2 cups chopped kale
1/4 cup chopped bell pepper
1/4 cup diced cucumber
1/4 cup sliced radish
1/4 cup fresh blueberries
1/4 cup diced avocado
2 tablespoons slivered almonds
2 tablespoons chopped fresh parsley
1 tablespoon chopped fresh mint
1 scallion, diced
1 cup shredded rotisserie chicken

FOR THE DRESSING
juice of 1/2 lime
2 tablespoons olive oil
1 teaspoon honey
1 teaspoon chia seeds
1/4 teaspoon salt
1/4 teaspoon pepper

1 Combine the bowl ingredients in a large bowl, and mix well.

2 Combine the dressing ingredients in a small bowl, and whisk until well combined. Set aside for 5 minutes to allow the chia seeds to absorb some of the liquid and thicken the mixture.

3 Stir the dressing once more and pour over the ingredients in the small bowl. Toss well to combine. Divide the mixture between two bowls and serve immediately.

Try this!
Vegan Vitality Superfood Salad

Replace the shredded chicken with 1 cup shelled edamame beans, and the honey with 1 teaspoon coconut or agave nectar. Finally, sprinkle 1 teaspoon hemp hearts over each bowl to garnish and increase the protein and omega fatty acids.

Vitality Berry Salad

Omit the radishes and add 1/4 cup fresh raspberries and 1/4 cup sliced strawberries. For the dressing, replace the lime juice with the juice of half a lemon, which will complement the flavor of the berries. To bring in one last touch of berry goodness, sprinkle 1/2 tablespoon dried, unsweetened cranberries over each bowl.

PER SERVING	
Calories	316
Protein	23g
Fat	16g
Carbohydrate	23g
Sugar	12g
Dietary fiber	10g
Vitamins	A, C
Minerals	calcium, iron

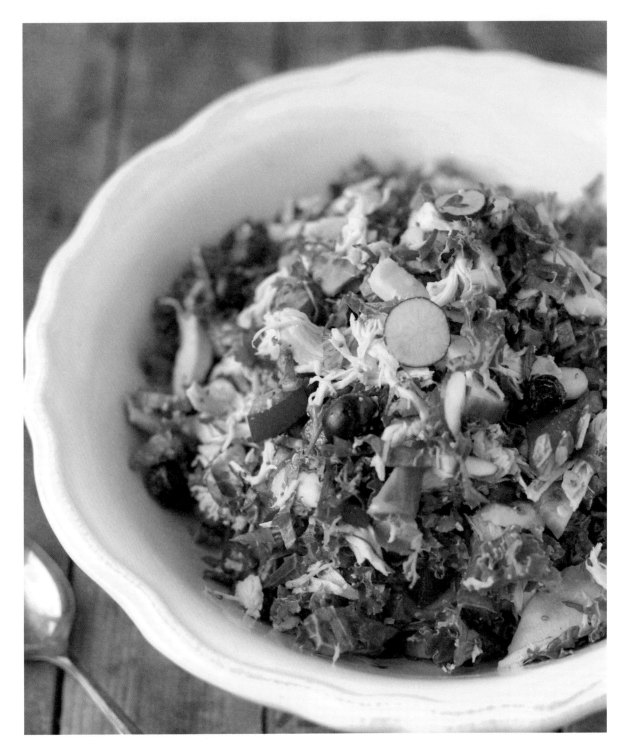

Zen Quinoa

SERVES · 1
PREPARATION TIME · 2 MINUTES
COOKING TIME · 10 MINUTES

1/2 teaspoon yellow curry powder
1/4 teaspoon garlic powder
1/4 teaspoon onion powder
1/4 teaspoon paprika
1/4 teaspoon salt
1/8 teaspoon freshly ground pepper
1/2 cup finely chopped broccoli florets
1/2 cup carrot, grated
1/4 cup sliced mushrooms
1 cup kale, torn into pieces
1/4 cup halved cherry tomatoes
1 lime, halved
1 egg
1/2 cup cooked quinoa
1/4 avocado, sliced
1/4 cup pea shoots

This recipe, inspired by a Hawaiian dish, uses curry and paprika flavors, with avocado and vegetables, to create a bowl that is balanced, healthy, and promotes a zenlike energy. The quinoa adds slow-releasing carbohydrates, while the egg provides protein and healthy fat.

1 In a small bowl mix together the curry powder, garlic powder, onion powder, paprika, and salt and pepper.

2 Heat a wok or saucepan over medium to high heat. When the wok is hot, add the broccoli, carrot, and mushrooms and a splash of water, then cook for 3 to 4 minutes, until the vegetables are tender.

3 Reduce the heat to medium and add the kale, tomatoes, and spice mix to the pan, and continue sautéing until the kale is wilted. If you are worried that the vegetables will stick or burn, add more water to the pan as needed.

4 Add the juice of half a lime to the kale. Crack the egg onto the top of the kale. Allow the egg to sit for a minute until it begins to cook, and then scramble the egg with the vegetables.

5 Place the cooked quinoa in a bowl. Top with the egg and vegetable mixture, and then garnish with the sliced avocado, pea shoots, and a squeeze of lime. Serve immediately.

PER SERVING	
Calories	329
Protein	17g
Fat	13g
Carbohydrate	50g
Sugar	7g
Dietary fiber	11g
Vitamins	A, C
Minerals	calcium, iron, magnesium, manganese

Try this!
Zen Fried Rice

Add vitamin B-rich brown rice to this bowl, which contributes complex carbohydrates and fiber, and makes for a healthy fried rice dish. Omit the paprika and yellow curry powder. Replace the quinoa with 1/2 cup of cooked brown rice. Add the rice to the pan with the vegetables and add 1 tablespoon of soy sauce (gluten-free if needed) with the egg. Once the egg is cooked, transfer the mixture to a bowl, garnish with the avocado and lime, and replace the pea shoots with 1/4 cup of chopped scallions.

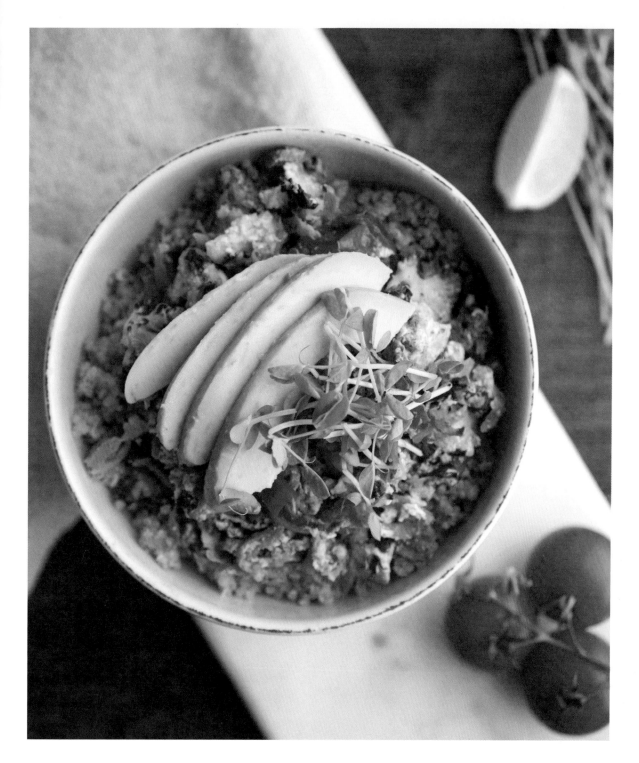

Mediterranean Chickpea Salad

SERVES · 1
PREPARATION TIME · 7 MINUTES

FOR THE DRESSING
Juice of 1/2 small lemon
1/8 teaspoon salt
1/8 teaspoon black pepper
1/2 tablespoon olive oil

FOR THE BOWL
1/2 cup halved cherry tomatoes
5 jumbo green olives, sliced
2 jarred artichokes
1/2 cup cucumber, diced
1/2 cup chickpeas, rinsed and drained
2 tablespoons jarred roasted red peppers or
   sun-dried tomatoes
Fresh parsley sprigs
1 tablespoon hummus
Lemon wedges

Light, fresh, and tasty, this bowl doesn't disappoint when it comes to health benefits. The Mediterranean-inspired ingredients contain powerful health-boosting nutrients for the cardiovascular and nervous system. Meanwhile, the chickpeas bring complex carbohydrates.

1 Whisk together the lemon juice, salt, pepper, and olive oil in a small bowl and set aside.

2 Arrange or layer the cherry tomatoes, olives, artichokes, cucumber, chickpeas, and roasted peppers or sun-dried tomatoes in a medium-sized bowl and garnish with the parsley.

3 Place the hummus in the center of the bowl. Drizzle with the dressing, and serve immediately with the lemon wedges on the side.

PER SERVING	
Calories	320
Protein	11g
Fat	18g
Carbohydrate	38g
Sugar	8g
Dietary fiber	10g
Vitamins	A, B_6, C
Minerals	calcium, iron, magnesium

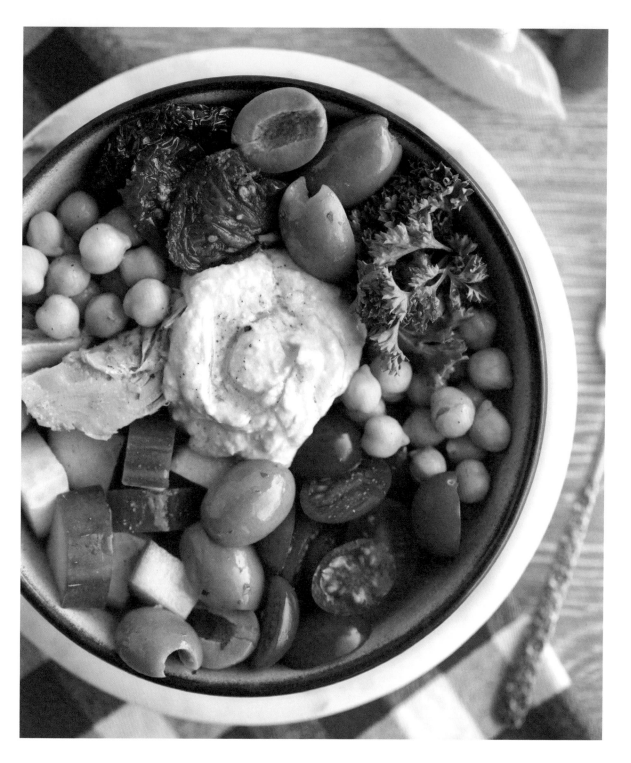

Try this!

Chilled Mediterranean Shrimp Pasta

This Italian-inspired recipe combines a light omega-rich dressing
with vitamin-rich raw vegetables, roasted peppers, artichokes,
protein-packed shrimp, and pasta that's loaded with complex
carbohydrates to provide long-lasting energy.

SERVES · 1
PREPARATION TIME · 7 MINUTES
COOKING TIME · 10 MINUTES

FOR THE BOWL
1/2 cup whole-grain or gluten-free pasta
1 teaspoon olive oil
1/2 cup halved cherry tomatoes
5 jumbo green olives, sliced
2 jarred artichokes
1/2 cup cucumber, diced
2 tablespoons jarred roasted red peppers or
   sun-dried tomatoes
6 large precooked wild shrimp, thawed if
   frozen
2 tablespoons finely chopped fresh parsley
sprig of fresh basil
Lemon wedges

FOR THE DRESSING
Juice of 1/2 small lemon
1/8 teaspoon salt
1/8 teaspoon black pepper
1/2 tablespoon olive oil

1 Cook the pasta according to the package instructions, drain,
and toss with the olive oil. Let cool, then chill in the refrigerator
until required.

2 Whisk together the lemon juice, salt, pepper, and olive oil
in a small bowl and set aside.

3 Arrange or layer the cherry tomatoes, olives, artichokes,
cucumber, and roasted peppers or sun-dried tomatoes in
a medium-sized bowl. Top with the shrimp and sprinkle
with the parsley.

4 Place the lemon and basil on top of the bowl. Drizzle with
the dressing, and serve immediately.

Try this!

Lemon & Artichoke Zucchini

Olive oil is known to benefit the skin, hair, and nails. It is
naturally high in unsaturated fats, particularly omega-9 fatty
acid. Here, it blends with lemon juice to create a light dressing
for a filling, fiber-rich, grain-free bowl featuring zucchini noodles
and a burst of vitamin C.

SERVES · 1
PREPARATION TIME · 10 MINUTES

FOR THE BOWL
1 large zucchini
1/4 teaspoon salt
5 jumbo green olives, sliced
2 jarred artichokes, chopped small
1/2 cup cucumber, diced
1/2 cup chickpeas, rinsed and drained
2 tablespoons finely chopped fresh parsley
1 tablespoon hummus
wedge of lemon

FOR THE DRESSING
Juice of 1/2 small lemon
1/8 teaspoon salt
1/8 teaspoon black pepper
1 tablespoon olive oil
1 teaspoon honey

1 Spiral the zucchini into "noodles." Place these in a medium-sized bowl and sprinkle with the salt.

2 Whisk together the dressing ingredients in a small bowl, until the honey is dissolved, and set aside.

3 Arrange or layer the olives, artichokes, cucumber, and chickpeas on top of the zucchini noodles and sprinkle with chopped parsley.

4 Pour over the dressing and mix well to combine, so that everything is coated with the dressing.

5 Top the bowl with the hummus, squeeze the lemon over it, and serve immediately.

Hawaiian Barbecue Tofu

SERVES · 1
PREPARATION TIME · 5 MINUTES
COOKING TIME · 10 MINUTES

1 teaspoon olive oil
3/4 cup cubed superfirm non-GMO organic
 tofu
1/4 teaspoon salt
1/8 teaspoon pepper
2 tablespoons barbecue sauce, divided
1/3 cup cooked brown rice, warmed
1/3 cup sliced fresh pineapple
1/4 cup sliced fresh mango
1/4 cup halved cherry tomatoes
1/2 cup sliced or spiralized zucchini
1 tablespoon sliced red onion
1 tablespoon crushed macadamia nuts

Enjoy fresh tropical flavors, with sweet and smoky barbecue sauce over tofu, pineapple, and mango, on a bed of brown rice. To top this nutrient-rich bowl, macadamia nuts—a Hawaiian staple—add magnesium, iron, and unsaturated fats.

1 Heat the olive oil in a nonstick skillet or frying pan over medium to high heat. Then add the tofu cubes, salt, and pepper. Sauté the cubes for 5 minutes, until they are brown and crisp on all sides.

2 Add 1 tablespoon of the barbecue sauce and 1 tablespoon of water to the hot pan, and stir to coat the cubes. Reduce the heat to low and stir for 1 to 2 minutes more, so the barbecue sauce coats the cubes.

3 Place the warmed brown rice in a bowl and top with the tofu. Arrange the pineapple, mango, tomatoes, zucchini, and red onion on top.

4 In a small bowl, whisk together the remaining 1 tablespoon of barbecue sauce and 1/2 tablespoon water, or heat them together in a small pan, if you prefer. Drizzle this mixture over the ingredients in the bowl. Sprinkle the macadamia nuts on top, and serve immediately.

PER SERVING	
Calories	403
Protein	18g
Fat	15g
Carbohydrate	53g
Sugar	25g
Dietary fiber	6g
Vitamins	C
Minerals	calcium, iron, magnesium

Try this!
Hawaiian Toasted Coconut Shrimp

Shrimp lightly coated with coconut adds fiber and protein to this bowl. Replace the tofu with 5 large deveined and peeled raw tiger shrimp. In a small bowl, combine 2 tablespoons of shredded unsweetened coconut, 1/2 tablespoon of all-purpose gluten-free flour, a pinch of salt and pepper, and 1/2 teaspoon of garlic powder. In another small bowl, combine 1 teaspoon of honey with 1 egg white and whisk until the honey is dissolved. Dip each shrimp in the honey-egg mixture. Then dredge the shrimp in the shredded coconut mixture to coat. Heat the olive oil in a pan. Fry the shrimp for 3 to 4 minutes on each side, until golden brown and slightly crispy (the shrimp should be completely pink and cooked through). Add the shrimp to the bowl with the warmed brown rice. Complete the recipe as directed, omitting the macadamia nuts.

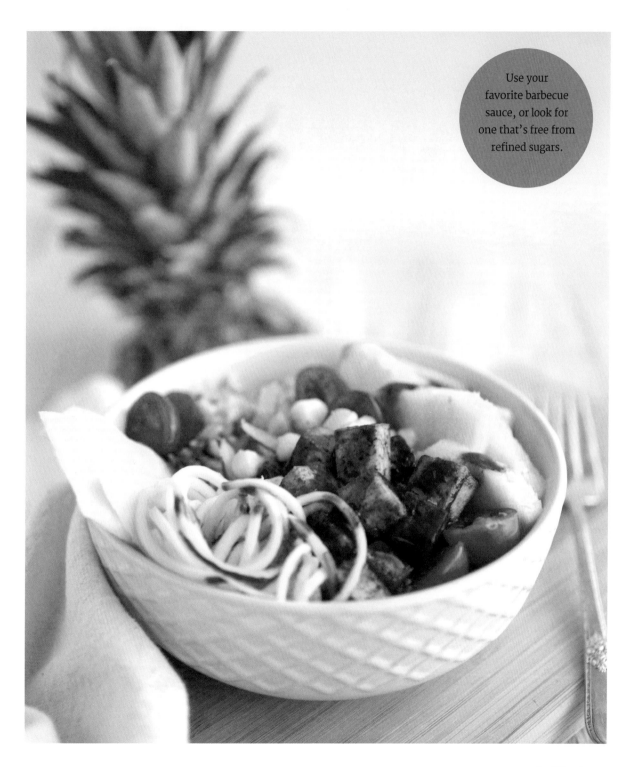

Use your favorite barbecue sauce, or look for one that's free from refined sugars.

California Chicken & Avocado

SERVES · 1
PREPARATION TIME · 10 MINUTES

FOR THE DRESSING
1 tablespoon pure maple syrup
1/2 tablespoon sesame tahini
1 tablespoon balsamic vinegar

FOR THE BOWL
2 cups of your favorite leafy greens (such as
    romaine, kale, spinach, and mixed greens)
1/4 cup pea shoots or sprouts
1/4 cup cherry tomatoes, halved
1/4 cup strawberries, sliced
1/4 avocado, pitted, sliced thick
2 1/2 ounces cooked chicken breast
1 strip cooked nitrate-free beef or pork bacon,
    chopped

In this bowl, leafy greens provide carbohydrates, fiber, and nutrients, and creamy avocado adds healthy omega-rich fats. A sweet and savory tahini, balsamic vinegar, and maple syrup dressing brings the bowl together.

1 Combine the maple syrup, tahini, vinegar, and 1 tablespoon water in a small bowl, and whisk until emulsified. Set aside.

2 Place the greens in a bowl, and then arrange the pea shoots, tomatoes, strawberries, avocado, chicken, and bacon on top.

3 Drizzle with the dressing, and serve immediately.

Try this!
California Edamame & Avocado

Edamame beans are an amazing source of plant-based protein, and they contain vitamins A and C. The Dijon mustard dressing is light and tangy. Replace the chicken and the bacon with 3/4 cup shelled edamame beans, and add them to the bowl with the pea shoots. Swap the tahini dressing for one made with 1/2 tablespoon Dijon mustard, 1/2 tablespoon raw honey, 1/2 tablespoon olive oil, 1/2 tablespoon apple cider vinegar, a pinch of salt and pepper, and 1 tablespoon of water, whisked together.

PER SERVING	
Calories	335
Protein	25g
Fat	13g
Carbohydrate	30g
Sugar	20g
Dietary fiber	7g
Vitamins	A, B_6, B_{12}, C
Minerals	calcium, iron, magnesium

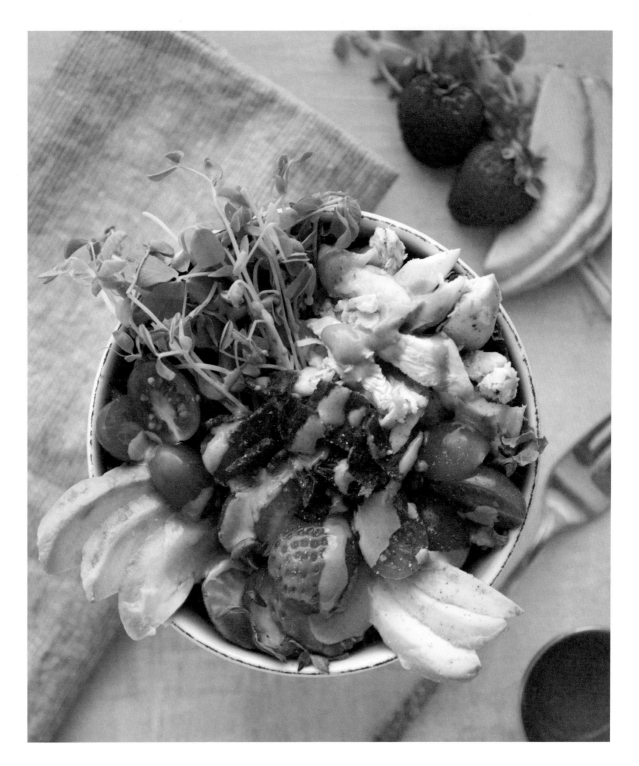

Steak Fajita Pasta

SERVES · 1
PREPARATION TIME · 15 MINUTES

FOR THE SAUCE
¼ teaspoon tapioca flour
1 tablespoon lime juice
1 teaspoon organic taco or fajita seasoning
  mix
1/8 teaspoon salt

FOR THE FAJITAS
1 teaspoon olive oil
1 clove garlic, crushed
¼ cup thinly sliced onion
3 ounces sirloin steak, sliced into strips
½ cup thinly sliced bell peppers
¾ cup cooked whole-grain or gluten-free
  pasta of choice
2 tablespoons cooked corn, warmed
¼ cup homemade or prepared salsa
2 tablespoons chopped fresh cilantro
2 lime wedges
1 tablespoon sour cream, or dairy-free sour
  cream, or crumbled feta, or shredded
  Cheddar cheese

Protein-packed steak and fiber-rich pasta add substance to this small but mighty bowl, which is topped with corn, cilantro, and lime. For even more freshness, make your own salsa with onion, tomatoes, cilantro, garlic, lime juice, salt, and pepper—just mix the ingredients together however you like them.

1 Combine the tapioca flour and 1 tablespoon cold water in a small bowl, and whisk until the tapioca is dissolved. Add the lime juice, seasoning mix, and salt, and whisk again until well incorporated. Set aside.

2 Heat the olive oil in a nonstick skillet or frying pan over medium to high heat. Add the crushed garlic and onion, and sauté for 2 minutes.

3 Add the steak and vegetables to the pan, and sauté. Add the sauce mixture. Continue to sauté for 5 minutes, until the sauce thickens slightly and glazes the steak and vegetables.

4 Once the steak is cooked as desired, and the peppers and onion have softened, remove the pan from the heat.

5 Place the pasta in a bowl, and add in the fajita steak mixture. Arrange the cooked corn, salsa, and cilantro on top. Then garnish with the lime wedges and sour cream or cheese. Serve immediately.

PER SERVING	
Calories	337
Protein	26g
Fat	12g
Carbohydrate	41g
Sugar	8g
Dietary fiber	3g
Vitamins	A, B_6, B_{12}, C
Minerals	calcium, iron

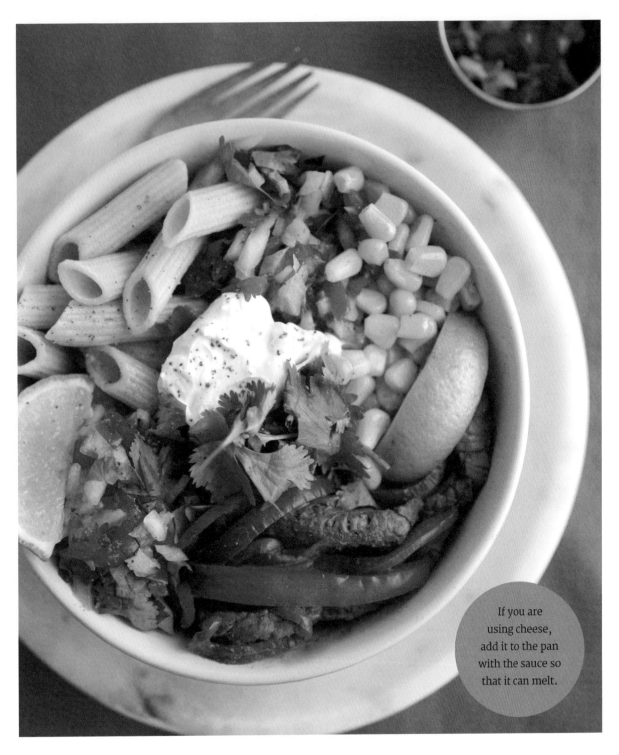

If you are using cheese, add it to the pan with the sauce so that it can melt.

Try this!

Beef Taco Salad

Go carb-free with this super easy and tasty taco salad bowl.
Carbohydrates aren't always necessary for a small meal,
especially if you are having a larger meal later in the day.

SERVES · 1
PREPARATION TIME · 15 MINUTES

FOR THE SAUCE
1/4 teaspoon tapioca flour
1 tablespoon lime juice
1 teaspoon organic taco or fajita
   seasoning mix
1/8 teaspoon salt

FOR THE FAJITAS
1 teaspoon olive oil
1 clove garlic, crushed
1/4 cup thinly sliced onion
3 ounces extralean ground beef
1/2 cup thinly sliced bell peppers
2 cups of shredded green leaf lettuce
2 tablespoons cooked corn, warmed
1/4 cup homemade or prepared salsa
2 tablespoons chopped fresh cilantro
2 lime wedges
1 tablespoon sour cream, or dairy-free
   sour cream, or crumbled feta, or
   shredded Cheddar cheese
2–3 corn tortilla chips, crushed

1 Combine the tapioca flour with 1 tablespoon cold water
in a small bowl and whisk until the tapioca is dissolved.
Add the lime juice, seasoning mix, and salt, and whisk
again until well incorporated. Set aside.

2 Heat olive oil in a nonstick skillet or frying pan over
medium to high heat. Add the crushed garlic and onions,
and sauté for 2 minutes.

3 Add the ground beef and bell peppers to the pan. Sauté the
ground beef and vegetables, and add the sauce mixture. Continue
to sauté for 5 minutes, until the sauce thickens slightly and glazes
the beef and vegetables.

4 Once the beef is cooked , and the peppers and onion have
softened, remove the skillet from the heat.

5 Place the lettuce in a bowl and add the beef and vegetable
mixture. Arrange the corn, salsa, and cilantro on top, and
then garnish with the lime wedges, sour cream or cheese,
and tortilla chips. Serve immediately.

Coconut-Lemongrass Vegetables

SERVES · 2
PREPARATION TIME · 2 MINUTES
COOKING TIME · 10 MINUTES

1 tablespoon red Thai curry paste
1 teaspoon sesame oil
1 teaspoon lemongrass paste or minced
  lemongrass
1 teaspoon ginger paste
1/2 cup full-fat canned coconut milk
2 small zucchini, spiralized or sliced with a
  mandoline
1 small sweet potato, peeled and spiralized,
  or sliced with a mandoline
1 small carrot, spiralized or sliced with a
  mandoline
1 small red bell pepper, julienned
1 tablespoon chopped fresh cilantro
1 tablespoon crushed peanuts or cashews
2 lime wedges

This Thai-inspired bowl combines the vitamins, minerals, and enzyme power of raw vegetables with fresh, spicy flavors and filling, healthy fats. It makes a healthy snack or lunch and supplies more nutrients than a daily multivitamin.

1 In a small saucepan heat the curry paste with the sesame oil over medium heat for 1 to 2 minutes. Stir in the lemongrass and ginger. Add the coconut milk and stir to combine. Bring the mixture to a simmer, then remove the pan from the heat.

2 Divide the sliced or spiralized vegetables between two bowls and pour the warm coconut-lemongrass sauce over the vegetables. Garnish with the cilantro, nuts, and lime wedges.

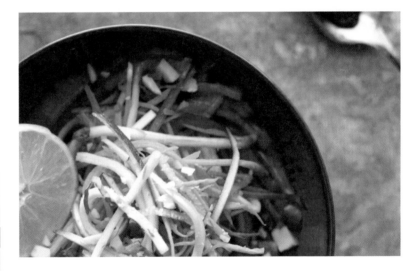

PER SERVING	
Calories	256
Protein	6g
Fat	14g
Carbohydrate	25g
Sugar	11g
Dietary fiber	7g
Vitamins	A, B, B$_6$, C
Minerals	calcium

Try this!
Coconut-Lemongrass Seared Tofu

Drizzle 1 cup cubed extrafirm tofu with coconut oil and sauté in a skillet or frying pan until brown and crispy on the outside. Stir the tofu into the finished sauce to coat, then divide the tofu and coconut sauce mixture evenly over the vegetables in each bowl and add the garnish.

Chicken & Quinoa Waldorf Salad

SERVES · 1
PREPARATION TIME · 10 MINUTES

3 ounces shredded cooked chicken breast
(use rotisserie chicken or baked
chicken breast)
1/4 cup diced apple
1/4 cup halved grapes
1/4 cup chopped celery
1/2 tablespoon organic mayonnaise
1 tablespoon plain Greek yogurt
1 teaspoon Dijon mustard
1/8 teaspoon salt
1/8 teaspoon pepper
1 1/2 cups fresh spinach
1/2 cup cooked quinoa
1 tablespoon chopped walnuts

Waldorf salad was created at the Waldorf Astoria hotel
in New York City. It's a delicious combination of crunchy,
juicy, fresh fruit and chicken in a creamy, rich dressing.
This version uses a lighter dressing made with Greek yogurt
and organic mayonnaise.

1 Shred or pull apart the chicken breast and combine it in a large bowl
with the apple, grapes, and celery.

2 In another small bowl combine the mayonnaise, yogurt, mustard,
salt, and pepper and mix well.

3 Add the yogurt sauce to the bowl with the chicken and mix to combine.

4 Add the spinach to another bowl and spoon the cooked quinoa on top.
Then top the quinoa with the chicken Waldorf mixture. Garnish with the
chopped walnuts and serve immediately.

Try this!
Creamy Chicken & Broccoli Pasta Salad

Keep the rich and creamy flavors of Waldorf Salad and add in some vitamin
C-rich broccoli. Replace the quinoa with 1/2 cup cooked whole-grain or gluten-
free pasta (bow tie or macaroni noodles will work well) for sustained energy.
Omit the apple, celery, and spinach, and add 1 cup chopped, raw broccoli
florets. To make the dressing, replace the Dijon mustard with 1 teaspoon of
white vinegar and the 1/2 tablespoon organic mayonnaise with an additional
1 tablespoon of Greek yogurt. Add 1 teaspoon of coconut palm sugar or cane
sugar to the dressing. Stir in 1 tablespoon of dried raisins.

PER SERVING	
Calories	359
Protein	25g
Fat	14g
Carbohydrate	33g
Sugar	7g
Dietary fiber	6g
Vitamins	A, B_6, B_{12}, C
Minerals	iron, magnesium

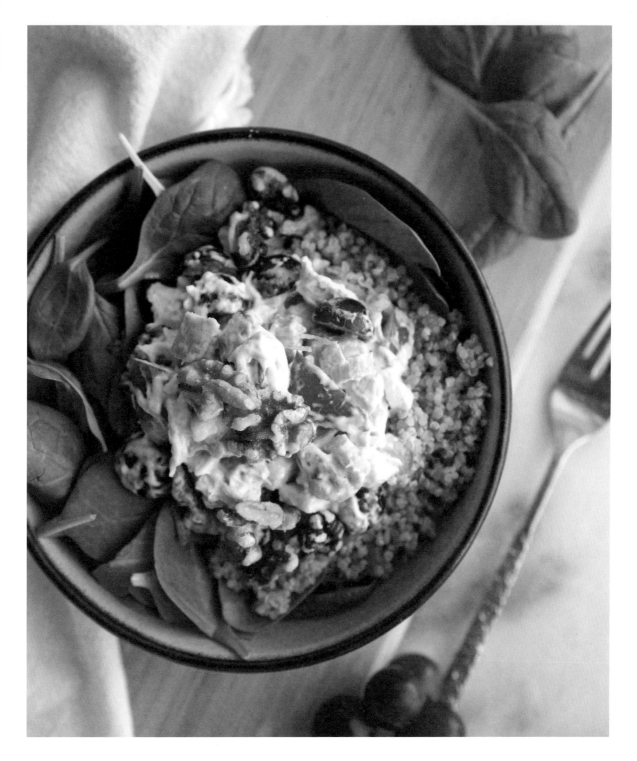

Shrimp Salad Roll with Peanut Sauce

SERVES · 1
PREPARATION TIME · 15 MINUTES

FOR THE BOWL
1/2 cup cooked white rice or brown rice
  vermicelli noodles
1 mini cucumber, sliced into thin ribbons
1/4 cup sliced red cabbage
2 tablespoons chopped scallion
1/4 cup chopped raw carrot
6 wild-caught tiger shrimp, peeled,
  deveined, and cooked
a few sprigs of fresh Thai basil
1 lime wedge

FOR THE SAUCE
1 tablespoon natural peanut butter
1 tablespoon lime juice
1/4 teaspoon sesame oil
1/4 teaspoon rice vinegar
1 teaspoon soy sauce
1 teaspoon honey
1 teaspoon fresh ginger (optional)

Traditional Vietnamese salad rolls are fresh, light, and tasty, but they require time and skill to make. This bowl combines all the flavors and nutrition of salad rolls in a quick and easy bowl. The light peanut sauce is perfect for drizzling over fresh vegetables, cooked shrimp, and silky rice noodles.

1 Place the rice vermicelli noodles in a bowl. Arrange the cucumber ribbons, cabbage, scallion, and chopped carrot on top. Add the cooked shrimp to the bowl.

2 Combine the peanut butter, lime juice, sesame oil, rice vinegar, soy sauce, honey, ginger, and 2 tablespoons of water in a small bowl and whisk until smooth, or combine in a small blender until smooth. Add more water, if you prefer a thinner consistency.

3 Drizzle the sauce over the bowl and garnish with the Thai basil leaves. Finish with a squeeze of fresh lime juice and serve immediately.

PER SERVING	
Calories	357
Protein	19g
Fat	10g
Carbohydrate	44g
Sugar	12g
Dietary fiber	5g
Vitamins	A, B_{12}, C, K
Minerals	magnesium, molybdenum, phosphorus, selenium

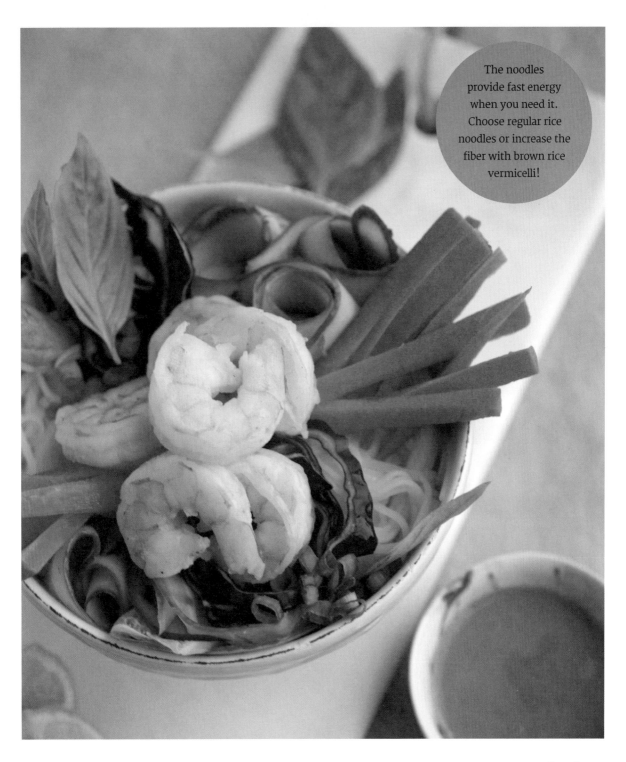

The noodles provide fast energy when you need it. Choose regular rice noodles or increase the fiber with brown rice vermicelli!

Try this!

Edamame, Avocado & Sesame Salad Roll

Enjoy a tasty vegan version of this Vietnamese classic. Edamame beans are a prime plant-based protein. The avocado introduces more omega-rich fats, and its creamy texture works well with the crunchy raw vegetables.

SERVES · 1
PREPARATION TIME · 15 MINUTES

FOR THE BOWL
1/2 cup cooked white rice or brown rice
    vermicelli noodles
1 mini cucumber, sliced in thin ribbons
1/4 cup sliced red cabbage
2 tablespoons chopped scallion
1/4 cup chopped raw carrot
1/4 cup of sliced avocado
1/2 cup cooked and shelled edamame
    beans
a few sprigs of fresh Thai basil
1 teaspoon toasted white or black sesame
    seeds
1 lime wedge

FOR THE SAUCE
1 tablespoon natural peanut butter
1 tablespoon lime juice
1/4 teaspoon sesame oil
1/4 teaspoon rice vinegar
1 teaspoon soy sauce
1 teaspoon coconut nectar
1 teaspoon fresh ginger (optional)

1 Place the rice vermicelli noodles in a bowl. Arrange or layer the cucumber, cabbage, scallion, carrot, and avocado on top. Add the edamame beans to the bowl.

2 Combine the peanut butter, lime juice, sesame oil, rice vinegar, soy sauce, coconut nectar, ginger, and 2 tablespoons of water in a small bowl and whisk until smooth, or combine in a small blender until smooth. Add more water if you prefer a thinner consistency.

3 Drizzle the sauce over the bowl and garnish with the Thai basil leaves and sesame seeds. Finish with a squeeze of fresh lime and serve immediately.

Try this!

Summer Fruit Salad Roll

Bring the fresh flavors of summer to this vegan bowl by adding ripe, seasonal fruit and a sweet tahini dressing. The fruit also offers plenty of antioxidants and fiber.

SERVES · 1
PREPARATION TIME · 15 MINUTES

FOR THE BOWL
1/2 cup cooked white rice or brown rice vermicelli noodles
1 mini cucumber, sliced in thin ribbons
2 tablespoons chopped scallion
1/4 cup chopped raw carrot
1/4 to 1/2 cup sliced fruit (e.g. strawberries, kiwi, mango)
1/4 cup sliced avocado
1/2 cup cooked and shelled edamame beans

FOR THE DRESSING
1 tablespoon pure maple syrup
1/2 tablespoon sesame tahini
1 tablespoon balsamic vinegar

1 Place the rice vermicelli noodles in a bowl.

2 Arrange or layer the cucumber, scallion, carrot, fruit, and avocado on top. Add the edamame beans to the bowl.

3 In a small bowl, whisk together the maple syrup, tahini, balsamic vinegar, and 1 tablespoon of water, until smooth.

4 Drizzle the dressing over the bowl and serve immediately.

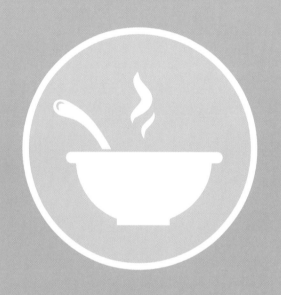

Big Bowls

When you want a hearty meal, you need a bowl that will do more than just fill you up. By including superfoods, high quality proteins, and complex carbohydrates, along with plenty of vegetables, you will get all the energy your body needs to see you through to your next meal.

Active Ingredients

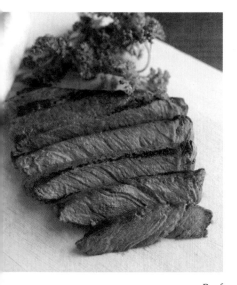

Beef

Beef

Origin Europe, Southeast Asia, and Africa
Food Family Bovine
Nutrients Fats, phosphorus, protein, selenium, zinc, vitamins B3, B6, B12, E
Power Properties This nutrient-dense protein has all the essential amino acids that support muscle growth and repair, as well as immune function. Beef from grass-fed animals contains CLA, a fatty acid that helps to heal inflammation and improves bone density, blood-sugar regulation, and muscle maintenance. Choose extralean sirloin or ground beef, as it has more protein per ounce.

Brown Rice

Origin Asia
Food Family Grasses
Nutrients Carbohydrates, copper, fiber, manganese, magnesium, phosphorus, selenium, vitamin B3
Power Properties This low glycemic index complex carbohydrate provides fiber and sustained energy. It supports digestion and disease prevention by keeping food moving smoothly through the digestive system. Plus, it contains selenium, which has been shown to reduce the risk of colon cancer. Whole-grain brown rice has all its nutritional layers, such as the germ and bran.

Kale

Origin Unknown
Food Family Cabbage
Nutrients Calcium, copper, fiber, manganese, vitamins A, B6, C, K
Power Properties This dense, leafy green is loaded with fiber and nutrients. It has been linked to improved eye and cardiovascular health and disease prevention. Just 1½ cups (100g) holds almost 1000 percent of the daily recommended intake of vitamin K, and 200 percent of the recommended daily intake of vitamins A and C.

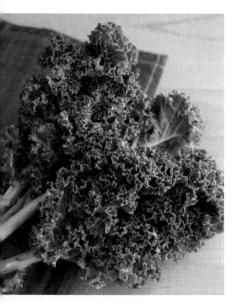

Kale

Plantain

Origin Southeast Asia

Food Family Plantaginaceae

Nutrients Carbohydrates, fiber, magnesium, potassium, vitamins A, B6, C

Power Properties Plantains may look like bananas, but they have different nutrients and fewer natural sugars. They have been known to help regulate digestion and immune function, provide antioxidants for disease prevention, and improve nervous system function. Buy plantains at the point of ripeness when they are yellow (not green), as they are slightly sweeter.

Quinoa

Origin The Andes region

Food Family Amaranthaceae

Nutrients Copper, fiber, folate, magnesium, manganese, phosphorus, zinc, vitamin B

Power Properties Quinoa is a low glycemic index complex carbohydrate that provides fiber and sustained energy for the body, thanks to its slow-releasing carbohydrate content. It also has plant-based proteins. When cooking quinoa, it's recommended to rinse it first and then cook it with vegetable, chicken, or beef broth to increase the flavor.

Salmon

Origin North Atlantic and Pacific

Food Family Salmonidae

Nutrients Omega-3 fatty acids, phosphorus, protein, selenium, vitamins B3, B6, B12, D

Power Properties The components in salmon include essential fatty acids, amino acids, vitamin D, and B vitamins. These nutrients promote nervous system, muscle, and skeletal health; immunity; and endurance. Its high fat content helps to prevent food cravings. Always choose wild or sustainably sourced fish.

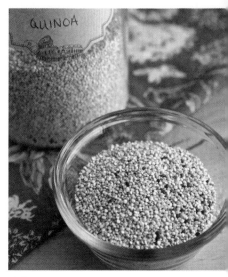

Quinoa

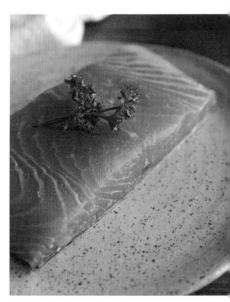

Salmon

Sweet Apple, Chicken & Coconut

SERVES · 1
PREPARATION TIME · 2 MINUTES
COOKING TIME · 20 MINUTES

1 teaspoon olive oil
3 ounces skinless, boneless chicken breast, diced
2 ounces skinless, boneless chicken thighs, diced
1/2 medium red apple, diced
1/4 teaspoon garlic powder
1/4 teaspoon onion powder
1/8 teaspoon salt
1/8 teaspoon pepper
1/4 cup halved cherry tomatoes
1 cup chopped kale
1/2 tablespoon pure maple syrup
1 tablespoon unsweetened shredded coconut, toasted if desired
3/4 cup cooked quinoa

Sometimes the most unlikely ingredients come together to create a powerful nutritional mix that benefits your health, as well as your taste buds. This recipe combines apples with kale, chicken, tomatoes, coconut, and sweet and savory seasonings. It makes a great meal in the colder months.

1 Heat the oil in a large skillet or frying pan over medium heat for 30 seconds, then add the chicken and sauté for 1 to 2 minutes.

2 Add the apple, garlic powder, onion powder, salt, and pepper, and cook for 5 to 7 minutes, until the chicken begins to brown and the apple softens. Add the cherry tomatoes, chopped kale, maple syrup, and 1 tablespoon of water.

3 Continue to sauté the ingredients for 5 minutes, until the chicken is cooked through and browned and the kale has wilted. Remove the skillet from heat.

4 Warm the quinoa on the stove for 1 to 2 minutes (or you can use the microwave), and place it in a medium-sized bowl. Place the chicken and kale mixture on top of the quinoa. Sprinkle with the shredded unsweetened coconut and serve immediately.

PER SERVING	
Calories	522
Protein	37g
Fat	17g
Carbohydrate	58g
Sugar	18g
Dietary fiber	12g
Vitamins	A, B$_6$, B$_{12}$, C
Minerals	calcium, iron, magnesium, manganese

Try this!
Sweet Apple & Bacon Warm Potato Salad

This is a healthier version of an indulgent warm potato salad. Replace the quinoa with 1 cup baby potatoes, halved and roasted in the oven at 400°F for 25 minutes, until fork-tender. Replace the chicken with 3 ounces of nitrate-free beef or pork bacon. Dice the bacon and sauté in a dry skillet or frying pan for 5 to 6 minutes, then drain on paper towel. Clean the pan, return to the heat, and add the olive oil, apple, and spices. Sauté for 3 to 4 minutes, then add the bacon. Combine the warm roasted potatoes in a bowl with the apple and bacon mixture. For added creaminess, stir 1/2 tablespoon of organic mayonnaise into the warm ingredients.

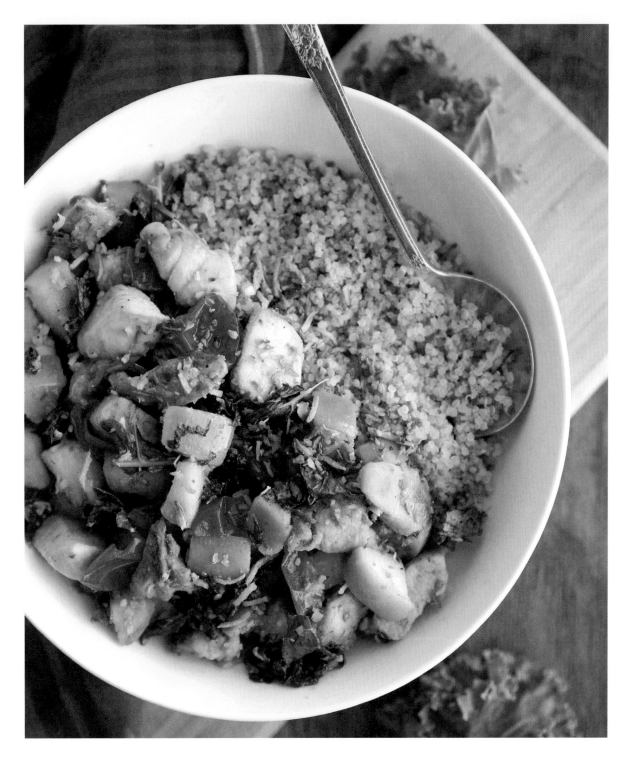

Pesto, Turkey & Kale Pasta

SERVES · 1
PREPARATION TIME · 10 MINUTES

1 cup torn kale
¼ teaspoon salt
1 cup cooked gluten-free or whole-grain
    penne pasta
2 tablespoons pesto
3 ounces baked or grilled turkey breast,
    chopped
2 sun-dried tomatoes, jarred in oil, chopped
sprig of fresh basil
pinch of black pepper
2 lemon wedges

If you are looking for fuel and flavor, this bowl is one to add to the list. The turkey, pasta, kale, and tomatoes are filling, healthy, and delicious. While pesto may seem indulgent, a little goes a long way, and it contains vitamins from the basil and unsaturated fats. Depending on the pasta used, this bowl can be gluten-free.

1 Place the kale in a large bowl, sprinkle it with the salt, and massage the leaves gently with your hands for 1 to 2 minutes, to soften them.

2 Place the cooked pasta in a separate bowl and stir in 1 tablespoon of the pesto to coat the pasta. Spoon the pasta on top of the kale.

3 In the same bowl, combine the turkey breast and the remaining pesto, and stir to coat.

4 Place the turkey on top of the kale and pasta. Add the chopped sun-dried tomatoes. Place a sprig of fresh basil in the middle of the bowl, sprinkle with a pinch of black pepper, and squeeze over the lemon wedges. Serve immediately.

PER SERVING	
Calories	513
Protein	35g
Fat	17g
Carbohydrate	56g
Sugar	4g
Dietary fiber	6g
Vitamins	A,B₃, B₆,C, K
Minerals	manganese, selenium

Try this!
Pesto, Turkey & Fig Quinoa

Lighten up the flavors and add a little sweetness by combining pesto and figs. Figs are a fantastic source of fiber, B vitamins, and minerals. Also, swap out pasta for quinoa, which bumps up the protein content. Replace the sun-dried tomatoes with 3 sliced fresh figs, the pasta with ¾ cup cooked quinoa, and the kale with spinach. Reduce the pesto to 1 tablespoon and use it to coat the turkey. Arrange or layer the spinach with the cooked quinoa, sliced figs, and pesto-coated turkey, and add a squeeze of lemon.
For an added flavor boost, drizzle 1 teaspoon balsamic reduction, or balsamic vinegar, and 1 teaspoon of olive oil, over the finished bowl.

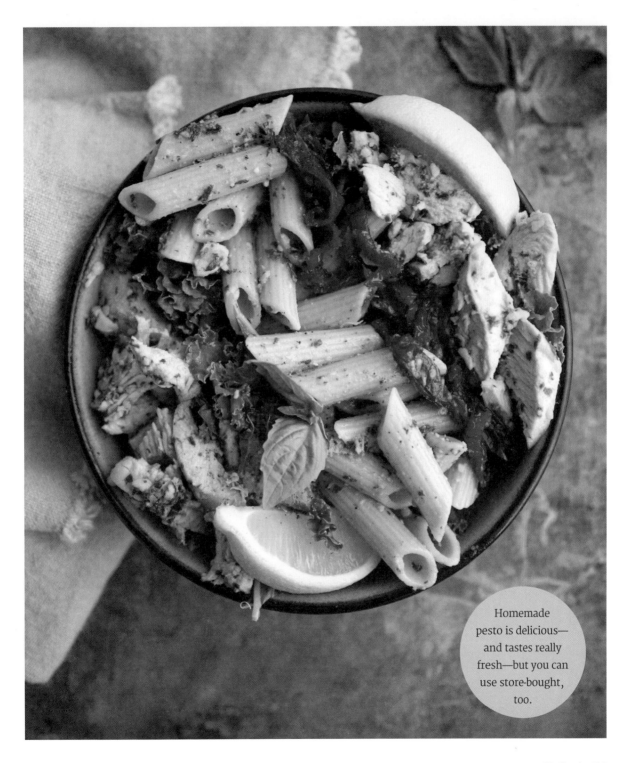

Homemade pesto is delicious—and tastes really fresh—but you can use store-bought, too.

Salmon & Kale Nicoise

SERVES · 1
PREPARATION TIME · 10 MINUTES
COOKING TIME · 30 MINUTES

FOR THE BOWL
1 cup baby potatoes, halved
1 small handful of green beans, cut and
    trimmed
3 cups torn red kale, washed and chopped
1/2 teaspoon sea salt
2 ounces smoked or cured salmon
1 hard-boiled egg, sliced
1/2 cup large olives, e.g. Castelvetrano

FOR THE DRESSING
1 tablespoon olive oil
2 tablespoons balsamic vinegar
1/4 teaspoon garlic powder
1/2 tablespoon Dijon mustard
1 teaspoon honey
pinch of salt
pinch of pepper

This combination of roasted potatoes, smoked salmon, olives, boiled egg, and green beans over a bed of kale is nothing less than perfection. Plus, it's loaded with powerful nutrients. Blanching the green beans seals in the flavor, nutrients, and color, while keeping a deliciously crunchy texture.

1 Preheat the oven to 400°F and line a baking pan with parchment paper. Place the potatoes in the prepared pan, cut side down, and roast for 15 minutes on one side, then turn them over and roast for another 10–15 minutes until done.

2 Meanwhile, heat 2 cups of water in a large saucepan and bring to a simmer over medium heat. Add the green beans and cook for 2 minutes. Then transfer to a colander and rinse under very cold water. Set the green beans aside.

3 Place the kale in a large bowl, sprinkle it with the salt, and gently massage the leaves with your hands for 1–2 minutes, to soften them.

4 Combine the dressing ingredients in a small bowl and whisk well.

5 Add the smoked salmon, egg, green beans, olives, and potatoes to the bowl with the kale. Drizzle with the dressing, then toss well to combine. Serve immediately, while the potatoes are still warm.

PER SERVING	
Calories	580
Protein	32g
Fat	26g
Carbohydrate	51g
Sugar	14g
Dietary fiber	10g
Vitamins	A, B$_{12}$, C, D, K
Minerals	calcium, iron, manganese

Try this!
Tuna, Spinach & Quinoa Nicoise

Speed up the preparation time by swapping out the roasted potatoes for quinoa, and increase the protein and omega-3 fatty acids by replacing the salmon with tuna. Cook 1/2 cup of dry quinoa with 1 cup of boiling water following the package instructions. Once cooked, fluff the quinoa with a fork and set it aside. Replace the kale with 3 cups of spinach and the smoked salmon with 3 ounces of sustainable canned tuna.

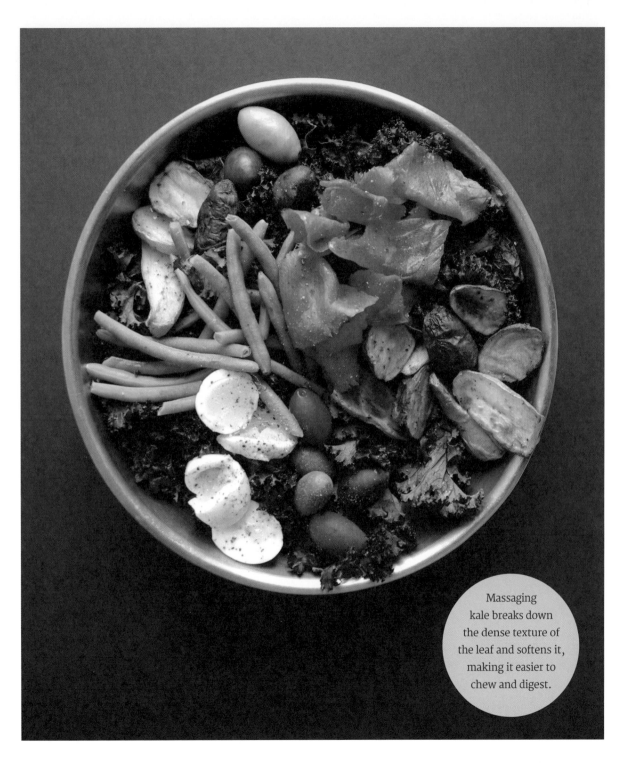

Massaging kale breaks down the dense texture of the leaf and softens it, making it easier to chew and digest.

Red Curry Dragon Bowl

SERVES · 2
PREPARATION TIME · 15 MINUTES
COOKING TIME · 15 MINUTES

FOR THE SAUCE
1 heaping tablespoon natural peanut butter
1/2 tablespoon tahini
1 tablespoon red Thai curry paste
1 tablespoon gluten-free soy sauce
1/4 teaspoon sesame oil
1 tablespoon coconut palm sugar
juice of 1 lime
1 clove garlic, crushed
1 teaspoon minced ginger or ginger paste
3/4 cup full-fat canned coconut milk

FOR THE BOWLS
2 x 3 ounce skinless, boneless chicken
   breasts, cut into small pieces
1 teaspoon coconut oil
1 red bell pepper, sliced
1 cup broccoli crowns, chopped
1/2 cup sugar snap peas
2 cups spinach
1 cup cooked brown rice
1/2 cup sliced red cabbage
1/2 cup shredded carrot
1/2 cup bean sprouts
1/4 cup fresh cilantro, chopped
2 tablespoons crushed peanuts

PER SERVING	
Calories	536
Protein	32g
Fat	28g
Carbohydrate	51g
Sugar	15g
Dietary fiber	9g
Vitamins	A, B_6, B_{12}, C, K
Minerals	iron, manganese, selenium

Dragon bowls are typically made with a bed of vitamin-rich spinach and warm brown rice topped with an array of vegetables and chicken. The red curry sauce contains healthy fats from the coconut milk, nut butter, and tahini, and delivers a fantastic hit of Thai-inspired flavors.

1 Combine all of the sauce ingredients, except the coconut milk, in a bowl and whisk until smooth. Set aside.

2 Place the coconut oil in a large skillet or frying pan, and cook over medium heat for 30 seconds to warm the oil. Add the chicken and cook, stirring frequently, for 10 minutes, until browned.

3 Place the sauce in another large saucepan or wok, and cook over medium-high heat until it comes to a simmer. Stir in the coconut milk and bring the sauce back to a simmer, then reduce the heat to medium. Add the bell pepper, broccoli, and snap peas to the sauce and cook for a few minutes, until the chicken has finished browning.

4 Add the browned chicken to the sauce and the vegetables. Cook for another 3 minutes, until the chicken is cooked through. Remove the pan from the heat.

5 Line two large bowls with the spinach and top with the warmed brown rice. Divide the chicken and vegetable curry between the bowls. Garnish with the raw cabbage, shredded carrot, bean sprouts, cilantro, and crushed peanuts. Serve immediately.

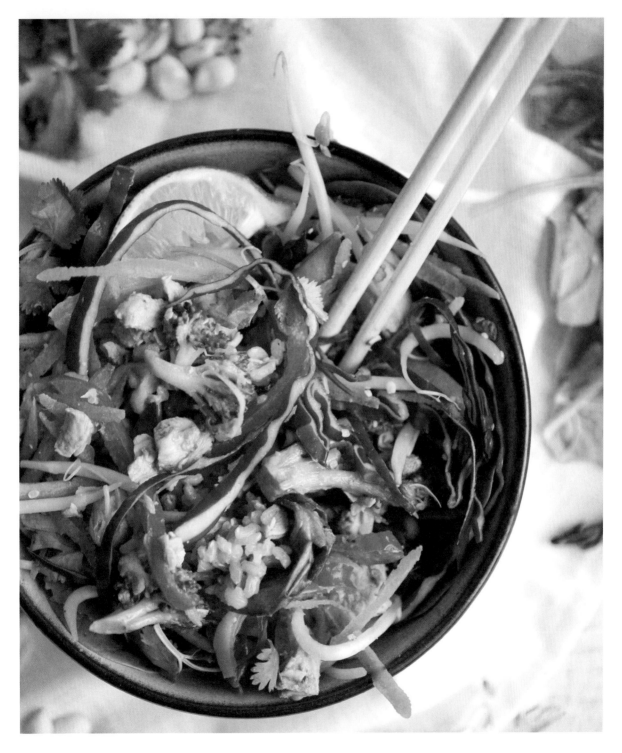

Try this!

Green Curry Dragon Bowl

Switch from red to green curry, and add some tropical flare and pistachio crunch. Pineapples are loaded with vitamin C, and add delicious juicy bites to the dish, while pistachios bring healthy fats to fill you up and nourish your body.

SERVES · 2
PREPARATION TIME · 15 MINUTES
COOKING TIME · 15 MINUTES

FOR THE SAUCE
1/2 tablespoon tahini
1 tablespoon green Thai curry paste
1 tablespoon gluten-free soy sauce
1/4 teaspoon sesame oil
1 tablespoon coconut palm sugar
juice of 1 lime
1 clove garlic, crushed
1 teaspoon minced ginger or ginger paste
3/4 cup full-fat canned coconut milk

FOR THE BOWLS
1 teaspoon coconut oil
2 x 3 ounce skinless, boneless chicken
  breasts, cut into small pieces
1 red bell pepper, sliced
1 cup broccoli crowns, chopped
1/2 cup diced fresh pineapple
2 cups spinach
1 cup cooked brown rice
1/2 cup sliced red cabbage
1/2 cup shredded carrot
1/2 cup bean sprouts
1/4 cup fresh cilantro, chopped
1/4 cup shelled raw pistachios

1 Combine all of the sauce ingredients, except the coconut milk, in a bowl and whisk until smooth. Set aside.

2 Place the coconut oil in a large skillet or frying pan, and cook over medium heat for 30 seconds to warm the oil. Add the chicken to the skillet and cook, stirring frequently, for 10 minutes, until browned.

3 Meanwhile, place the sauce in another large saucepan or wok, and cook over medium-high heat until it comes to a simmer. Stir in the coconut milk, bring the sauce back to a simmer, then reduce the heat to medium. Add the bell pepper, broccoli, and pineapple to the sauce and cook for a few minutes, until the chicken has finished browning.

4 Add the browned chicken to the sauce and the vegetables. Cook for another 3 minutes, until the chicken is cooked through. Remove the pan from the heat.

5 Line two large bowls with the spinach, and top with the warmed, cooked brown rice. Divide the chicken and vegetable curry between the bowls. Garnish with the cabbage, carrot, bean sprouts, cilantro, and pistachios. Serve immediately.

Try this!

Vegan Sweet Potato Dragon Bowl

This filling dragon bowl is packed with plant proteins. The sweet potato contains fiber and vitamin A, along with complex carbohydrates for sustained energy. Swapping out the chicken for edamame beans keeps the protein up and adds minerals.

SERVES · 2
PREPARATION TIME · 15 MINUTES
COOKING TIME · 15 MINUTES

FOR THE SAUCE
1 heaping tablespoon natural peanut
   butter
1/2 tablespoon tahini
1 tablespoon red Thai curry paste
1 tablespoon gluten-free soy sauce
1/4 teaspoon sesame oil
1 tablespoon coconut palm sugar
juice of 1 lime
1 clove garlic, crushed
1 teaspoon minced ginger or ginger paste
3/4 cup full-fat canned coconut milk

FOR THE BOWLS
1 teaspoon coconut oil
1 1/2 cups of cubed sweet potato, cut into
   1 in. cubes
1/2 cup sugar snap peas
1 cup broccoli crowns, chopped
1 red bell pepper, sliced
1 cup shelled edamame beans
2 cups spinach
1/2 cup sliced red cabbage
1/2 cup shredded carrot
1/2 cup bean sprouts
1/4 cup fresh cilantro, chopped
2 tablespoons crushed peanuts
1 lime, halved

1 Combine all of the sauce ingredients, except the coconut milk, in a bowl and whisk until smooth. Set aside.

2 Place the coconut oil in a large skillet or frying pan, and cook over medium heat for 30 seconds to warm the oil. Add the sweet potato cubes and cook, stirring frequently, for 5 minutes, until browned.

3 Meanwhile, place the sauce in another large saucepan or wok, and cook over medium-high heat until it comes to a simmer. Stir in the coconut milk, bring the sauce back to a simmer, then reduce the heat to medium.

4 Add the sweet potato to the sauce and cook for 7 minutes, then add the sugar snap peas, broccoli, and bell pepper. Cook for 5 minutes, then add the edamame beans. Simmer for 3–4 minutes, until the sweet potatoes are fork-tender. Remove the pan from the heat.

5 Line two large bowls with the spinach and divide the vegetable curry between the bowls. Garnish with the raw cabbage, carrot, bean sprouts, cilantro, and crushed peanuts. Squeeze 1/2 a lime over each bowl. Serve immediately.

Orange, Beef & Broccoli Noodles

SERVES · 2
PREPARATION TIME · 25 MINUTES
COOKING TIME · 25 MINUTES

FOR THE SAUCE
1 tablespoon tapioca flour
2 tablespoons rice vinegar
1/4 cup gluten-free soy sauce
3 tablespoons orange juice
2 tablespoons coconut palm sugar

FOR THE BOWLS
1/2 tablespoon olive oil
1 clove garlic, crushed
8 ounces beef sirloin, cut into strips
1 1/2 cups broccoli florets
1 red bell pepper, cut into strips
1/2 navel orange, cut into chunks
3 ounces dry soba (buckwheat) noodles,
    cooked and kept hot
1/2 teaspoon orange zest
1/2 teaspoon roasted sesame seeds

Sometimes there's nothing more satisfying than a stir-fry. These bowls contain vitamin-rich orange, which adds natural sweetness and a delicious citrus flavor to the beef and broccoli. These bowls taste even better the next day, when the flavors have had time to intensify.

1 Prepare the sauce by whisking together the tapioca flour and 3 tablespoons cold water in a bowl, until the tapioca is dissolved. Add the remaining ingredients and whisk until the coconut sugar is dissolved. Set aside.

2 Heat the olive oil in a large wok or saucepan over medium-high heat. Add the beef strips and crushed garlic. Sauté for 1–2 minutes, to slightly brown the beef. Pour in the sauce and reduce the heat to medium, until the sauce starts to thicken and bubble.

3 Add in the broccoli and bell pepper, and stir-fry with the sauce. Cover the wok or pan with a lid, and let the vegetables continue to cook with the beef and sauce. Reduce the heat to low, add the chopped orange, and stir to coat the orange with the sauce.

4 Divide the noodles between two bowls, top with the beef mixture, and garnish with orange zest and sesame seeds. Serve immediately.

PER SERVING	
Calories	484
Protein	40g
Fat	9g
Carbohydrate	65g
Sugar	18g
Dietary fiber	4g
Vitamins	A, B$_6$, B$_{12}$, C, K
Minerals	iron, magnesium

Try this!
Ginger & Lime Shrimp Fried Rice

For a change of flavor and texture, use a leaner protein—shrimp—and replace the noodles with rice. You will need 8 ounces of raw, peeled, wild shrimp and 1 1/2 cups cooked brown rice. Replace the orange juice with 2 tablespoons of lime juice and 1 teaspoon of grated fresh ginger, and the diced orange with 3/4 cup of thinly sliced carrot. Sauté the garlic, broccoli, pepper, and carrot for 4 to 5 minutes, until softened, then add the shrimp and the sauce. As the sauce begins to thicken, reduce the heat to medium, and stir the ingredients together. As soon as the shrimp is cooked (about 3 to 4 minutes), turn off the heat. Divide the warm rice between two bowls, then top with the shrimp. Garnish with sesame seeds and lime juice, but omit the orange zest.

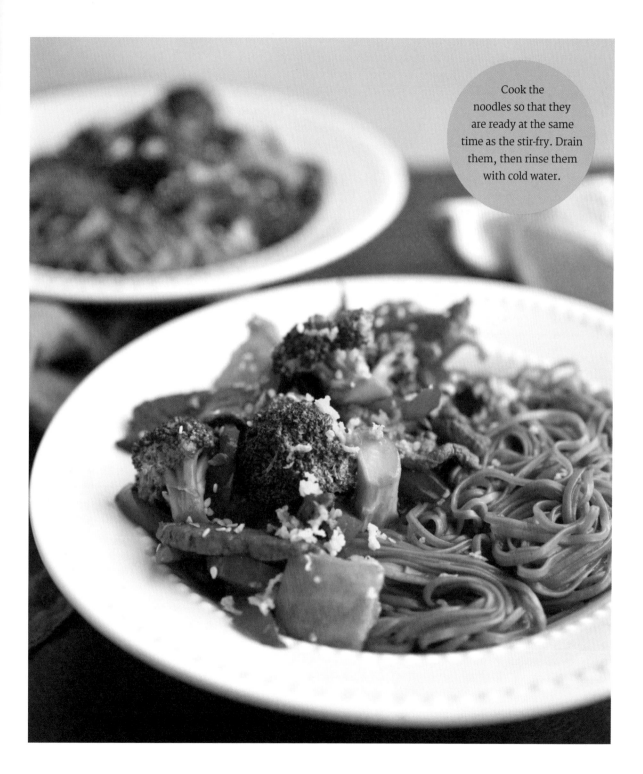

Cook the noodles so that they are ready at the same time as the stir-fry. Drain them, then rinse them with cold water.

Seared Ahi Tuna, Citrus & Quinoa

SERVES · 1
PREPARATION TIME · 10 MINUTES
COOKING TIME · 5 MINUTES

FOR THE DRESSING
1/2 cup fresh cilantro
1/2 clove garlic
juice of 1/2 lime
1 tablespoon finely diced fresh pineapple
1 teaspoon honey
1/2 tablespoon olive oil
pinch of salt
pinch of pepper

FOR THE BOWL
1 tablespoon roasted sesame seeds
1/8 teaspoon salt
1/8 teaspoon pepper
4 ounces raw sushi-grade yellow-fin ahi tuna
    steak
1 teaspoon olive oil, divided
3/4 cup cooked quinoa
1 cup arugula
1/2 orange, peeled and sliced
1/3 cup sliced grapefruit
1/2 avocado, peeled, pitted, and sliced
1/2 cup sliced cucumber
1/4 cup cherry tomatoes, halved

The citrus flavors of grapefruit and orange blend wonderfully with seared sesame-crusted ahi tuna over a bed of spicy arugula and carbohydrate-rich quinoa. A cilantro-garlic dressing provides a hefty dose of vitamin A, along with a tang and sweetness to balance the flavors.

1 Combine the dressing ingredients in a small food processor and pulse until emulsified and mostly smooth (leave some larger pieces of cilantro). Chill until required.

2 Combine the roasted sesame seeds, salt, and pepper in a bowl. Brush the tuna steak with 1/2 teaspoon olive oil, then press it into the sesame seeds to coat the outside. Turn it over to coat the other side.

3 Heat a skillet or frying pan over medium heat and add the remaining 1/2 teaspoon of olive oil. When the oil is hot, and the pan is very hot, add the tuna and sear for 1 to 2 minutes on one side. Turn the steak over, and sear for 1 to 2 minutes on the other side. Using tongs to hold the steak, sear the edges for 15 to 30 seconds on each side. Set the steak on a cutting board to rest.

4 Combine the quinoa and arugula in a bowl. Arrange or layer the orange, grapefruit, avocado, cucumber, and tomatoes on top. Cut the tuna into strips and place them on top of the bowl. Drizzle with the cilantro-garlic dressing. Serve immediately.

PER SERVING	
Calories	570
Protein	39g
Fat	10g
Carbohydrate	62g
Sugar	10g
Dietary fiber	10g
Vitamins	A, B$_3$, B$_6$, B$_{12}$, C
Minerals	iron, magnesium, selenium

Try this!
Mexican Seared Ahi Tuna

Keep the vitamin-rich tuna, slow energy-releasing quinoa, and arugula while enjoying some Mexican flavors. Coat the tuna with 1 teaspoon organic taco seasoning, and omit the pineapple from the dressing. Replace the grapefruit, orange, and cucumber with 1/4 cup corn kernels and 2 tablespoons of warmed black beans. Finish the bowl with a squeeze of lime and a dollop of sour cream and salsa.

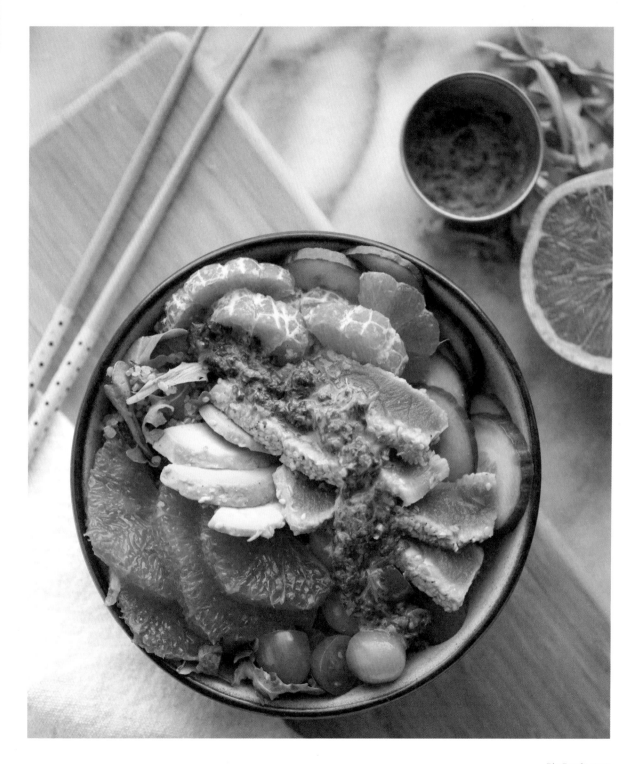

Pulled Cuban Chicken

SERVES · 1
PREPARATION TIME · 5 MINUTES
COOKING TIME 15 MINUTES

FOR THE GARNISH
1/4 cup avocado
1 tablespoon salsa verde (green salsa)
squeeze of fresh lime juice
salt and black pepper
1 teaspoon coconut oil
1/2 cup sliced plantain
pinch of ground cinnamon
pinch of coconut palm sugar

FOR THE BOWL
1/4 cup sliced onion
1 roma tomato, diced
1 small clove garlic, crushed
1/2 cup shredded cooked chicken
pinch of cayenne pepper
pinch of chili powder
pinch of red pepper flakes
pinch of ground cumin
pinch of ground cloves
salt and black pepper
1/2 cup cooked brown rice, warmed
1/4 cup cooked black beans, warmed
2 sprigs fresh cilantro
1 lime wedge

PER SERVING	
Calories	590
Protein	37g
Fat	18g
Carbohydrate	74g
Sugar	16g
Dietary fiber	14g
Vitamins	A, B$_6$, B$_{12}$, C
Minerals	iron, magnesium, manganese

Cuban-inspired flavors unite in this hearty bowl. Lightly fried plantain—a staple Cuban ingredient—is the star, and blends well with the brown rice and black beans. Additional flavors come from shredded chicken and avocado mashed with salsa verde. Cilantro and lime create a light and fresh finish.

1 Combine the avocado, salsa, lime juice, and salt in a bowl, and mash with a fork until mostly smooth. Chill until required.

2 Warm the coconut oil in a large nonstick skillet or frying pan over medium-high heat for 30 seconds, then add the plantain. Add the salt, pepper, cinnamon, and sugar, and cook for 2 minutes. Turn the plantain over and fry for another 2 minutes. Remove the plantain from the pan and drain on paper towels.

3 Reduce the heat to medium and add 1 tablespoon of water to the pan to de-glaze it. Add the onion, tomato, garlic, and chicken and sauté for 1 to 2 minutes, until the vegetables begin to soften.

4 Sprinkle the cayenne pepper, chili powder, red pepper flakes, cumin, cloves, salt, and pepper over the vegetables in the pan and sauté for 5 to 7 minutes, until the tomatoes are soft and the juices run into the rest of the ingredients. Reduce the heat to low.

5 Place the warmed rice and beans in the bottom of a bowl, then place the plantain slices on top, followed by the chicken mixture. Top with the mashed avocado, and garnish with the cilantro and a squeeze of the lime wedge. Serve immediately.

Try this!
Spicy Cuban Pinto Beans

Pinto beans are packed with protein, rich in magnesium, iron, and vitamin B$_6$, and are a great vegan alternative to the chicken. Increasing the red pepper flakes will add some more heat. Replace the chicken with 1/2 cup cooked pinto beans and add them to the pan with the tomato and onion. Add 1/8 teaspoon of red pepper flakes with the rest of the spices. Garnish the bowl with 1/8 teaspoon of cinnamon.

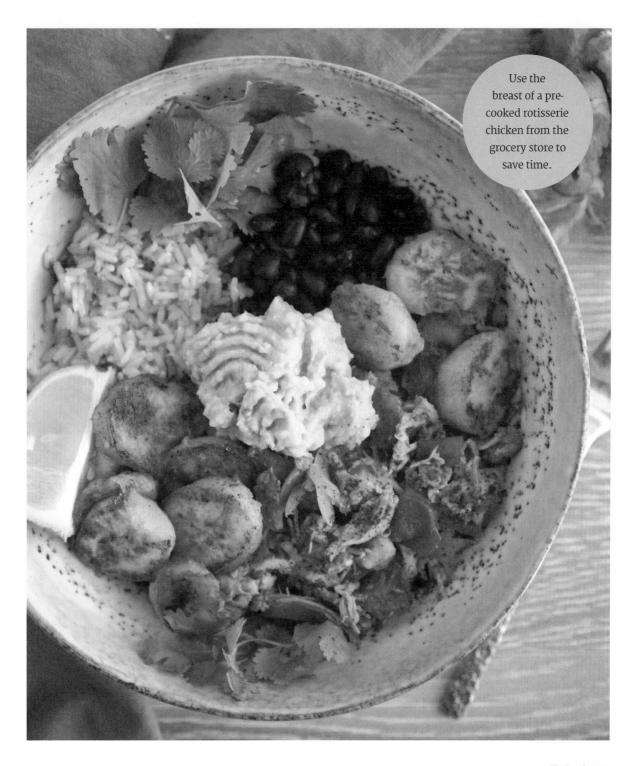

Use the breast of a pre-cooked rotisserie chicken from the grocery store to save time.

Slow-Cooked Thai Chicken Curry

SERVES · 4
PREPARATION TIME · 15 MINUTES
COOKING TIME · 4 HOURS

FOR THE SAUCE
1 (15-ounce) can light coconut milk
1/2 cup raw cashews
1 heaping tablespoon Thai green curry paste
5-6 Kaffir lime leaves
1 tablespoon lime juice
1 teaspoon minced garlic
1 teaspoon minced ginger root
1/4 cup fresh cilantro

FOR THE BOWL
4 (4 ounce) boneless chicken breasts
1 small yellow onion, diced
2 bell peppers, sliced
1 medium carrot, sliced
1 cup green beans, chopped
1 (15-ounce) can chickpeas, drained
  and rinsed
1/4 cup chopped fresh cilantro
4 Kaffir lime leaves
1 tablespoon lime juice
1 tablespoon sesame oil
1/4 cup pistachios
1/4 cup crushed cashews

PER SERVING	
Calories	560
Protein	41g
Fat	35g
Carbohydrate	36g
Sugar	12g
Dietary fiber	9g
Vitamins	A, B$_6$, B$_{12}$, C
Minerals	iron, magnesium

This recipe might take a long time, but don't be fooled —it's easy to put together. As it cooks, the chicken, carrots, onions, peppers, and green beans are wrapped in a rich, velvety, curry sauce. It creates an unbelievably tasty, tender, and warming stew.

1 Combine the sauce ingredients in a high-speed blender and blend until smooth.

2 Skin the chicken breasts if necessary, and cut the flesh into pieces. Combine the chicken, onion, peppers, and carrots in the slow cooker. Add the sauce and toss to coat. Cook on high for 3 hours, stirring every 30 minutes.

3 Add the green beans and chickpeas, and cook for another 1 hour.

4 Divide the curry between four bowls and top with the chopped cilantro, lime leaves, lime juice, sesame oil, and pistachios. Garnish with the chopped cashews and serve immediately.

Try this!
Slow-Cooked Butter Chicken

Change the spices in the sauce to switch to a tasty Indian curry. Use coconut milk and cashews for creaminess, along with aromatic spices, including turmeric, which is a natural anti-inflammatory and great for your joints. Replace the Thai green curry paste, Kaffir lime leaves, lime juice, and cilantro in the sauce with 1 teaspoon yellow curry powder, 1 teaspoon red Thai curry paste, 1 heaping tablespoon garam masala, 1 teaspoon ground turmeric, 1 teaspoon cayenne pepper, 1/4 teaspoon salt, and one 6-ounce can of tomato paste. Omit the chickpeas. Divide 2 cups cooked brown rice between the four bowls and then divide the curry between them. Omit the lime leaves, lime juice, and sesame oil from the garnish.

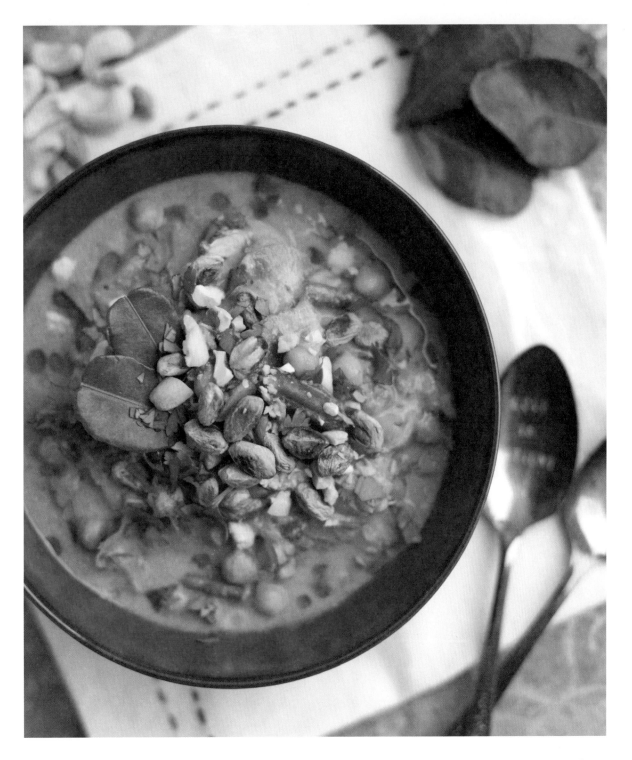

Mojito Shrimp & Zucchini

SERVES · 2
PREPARATION TIME · 35 MINUTES
COOKING TIME · 5 MINUTES

FOR THE MARINADE AND DRESSING
1 tablespoon canola oil
1 tablespoon honey
juice of 2 limes
¼ cup chopped fresh mint
¼ cup chopped fresh cilantro
¼ teaspoon salt
¼ teaspoon pepper

FOR THE BOWLS
14 large sustainable wild-caught shrimp, raw
1 red bell pepper, julienned
1 yellow bell pepper, julienned
¼ cup sliced red onion
1 avocado, pitted, peeled, and diced
2 large zucchini, spiralized or sliced into
   pasta strips with a mandoline, or cubed
salt
pepper

When it comes to vegetable power, this bowl has it all. Strips of zucchini make a nutritious base for wild-caught shrimp, and the refreshing mojito dressing is full of vitamin C. While it doesn't contain whole grains, this bowl does have energy-boosting carbohydrates and is easy on the digestive system.

1 Combine the dressing ingredients in a bowl and whisk together. Divide between two bowls, and set one bowl aside. Add the shrimp to the dressing in the remaining bowl, toss to coat, and place in the fridge to marinate.

2 Combine the peppers, onion, avocado, and reserved dressing in a bowl, and toss to coat. Chill for 30 minutes to marinate.

3 Meanwhile, divide the zucchini between two bowls and season lightly with salt and pepper.

4 Grill the shrimp for 2 to 3 minutes, until cooked, or sauté in a hot pan for 4 to 5 minutes.

5 Combine the cooked shrimp with the chilled, marinated vegetables and toss to combine so that everything is coated with the dressing. Divide the vegetable and shrimp mixture between the bowls of zucchini. Serve immediately.

PER SERVING	
Calories	421
Protein	31g
Fat	20g
Carbohydrate	37g
Sugar	21g
Dietary fiber	12g
Vitamins	A, B₁₂, C
Minerals	copper, manganese, phosphorus, selenium

Try this!
Mojito Shrimp Pasta Salad

Need an even bigger bowl, or more slow-releasing complex carbohydrates for long-lasting energy in your day? Replace the zucchini with chilled, gluten-free, or whole-grain pasta noodles, and you'll feel full and energized for hours. Toss 2 cups of cooked and drained pasta with 1 teaspoon of olive oil to prevent it from sticking, then chill with the shrimp and vegetables. When you are ready to cook the shrimp, divide the pasta between two bowls and complete the recipe as directed.

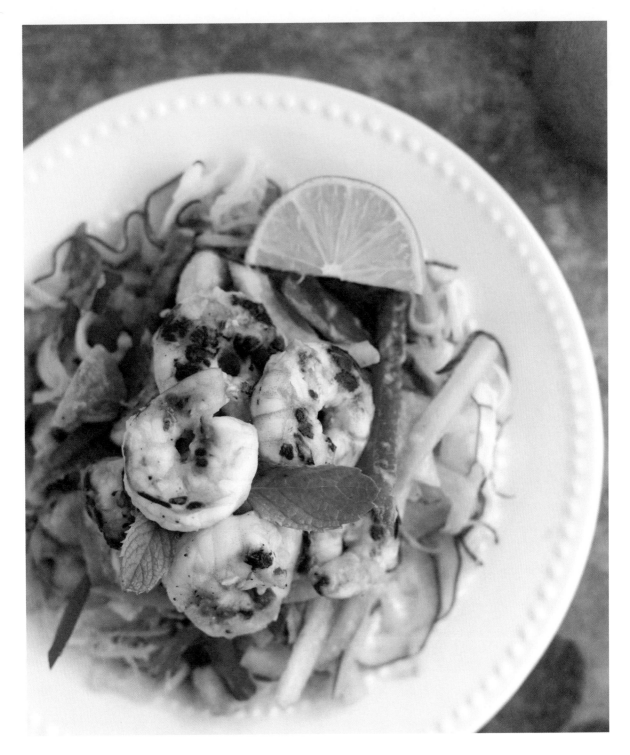

Treat Bowls

Making a treat bowl that contains vitamins, minerals, and proteins, and tastes sweet and creamy may sound impossible—but these recipes prove it's easy when you know how. By choosing ingredients that are naturally sweet, antioxidant-rich, and which also supply a delicious creaminess, you can enjoy both a healthy bowl and a sumptuous treat.

Active Ingredients

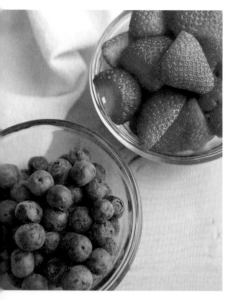

Berries

Berries
Origin Various
Food Family Various
Nutrients Carbohydrates, copper, fiber, manganese, vitamins C and K
Power Properties Berries, such as blueberries, raspberries, strawberries, and blackberries are naturally sweet and juicy. Plus, they are loaded with nutrients. Berries are crammed with antioxidants that help combat disease and improve immunity, plus they contain fiber to enhance digestive function, fill you up, and satisfy cravings.

Chocolate
Origin The Americas
Food Family Theobroma
Nutrients Calcium, copper, fats, iron, magnesium, manganese
Power Properties Sweet, rich, and decadent, chocolate has always had its place in the treat category. Chocolate that contains at least 70 percent cocoa solids, few added sugars, and no dairy products is high in antioxidants and minerals, and makes a better choice than chocolate that is loaded with sugar and milk products. Choose organic, naturally sweetened chocolate with a minimum of 70 percent cocoa.

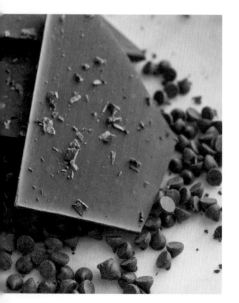

Chocolate

Coconut Cream
Origin Australia and India
Food Family Palm Tree
Nutrients Medium chain diglycerides, fiber, iron, magnesium
Power Properties Coconut cream is the perfect alternative to regular cream. It can be transformed into a topping, whipped (just like dairy cream), or used to make nondairy ice cream. Its fats have been shown to improve energy, plus their antimicrobial compounds help support your immune system. The fiber in coconut cream stimulates digestion, and the minerals provide an added health boost.

Coconut Yogurt

Origin Unknown, produced in several countries
Food Family Palm Tree
Nutrients Calcium, medium chain diglycerides, fiber, iron, magnesium, vitamin B12 and D
Power Properties Coconut yogurt is made from coconut milk and is a substitute for dairy yogurt. While it does not have the same amount of protein as Greek yogurt, it does contain nutrients. For these recipes, use a plain, unsweetened variety and add your own natural sweeteners, such as honey or coconut nectar.

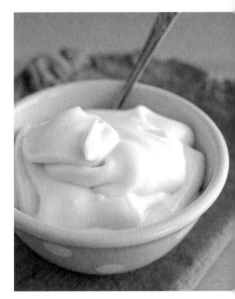

Coconut yogurt

Honey

Origin Asia
Food Family Various
Nutrients Calcium, carbohydrates, copper, iron, magnesium, manganese, trace amounts of vitamins B1, B2, B3, B5, B6
Power Properties Honey is a top choice when you need an unrefined, unprocessed natural sweetener. Not only does it contain vitamins and minerals, it also has natural antibacterial properties. Choose raw, unpasteurized honey, as the pasteurization process can eliminate the beneficial trace minerals.

Silken Tofu

Origin China
Food Family Legume
Nutrients Calcium, copper, manganese, omega essential fatty acids phosphorus, protein, selenium
Power Properties When it comes to plant-based protein, tofu is a top-notch choice. Made from soy milk, it has been linked to improved cardiovascular health. Silken tofu has a softer consistency than regular tofu. It can be used to create a creamy base similar to yogurt, and blends well with fruits and sweeteners. Buy an unsweetened, non-GMO variety.

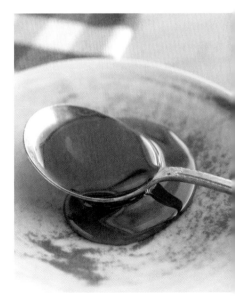

Honey

Lemon, Kiwifruit & Coconut Cream "Pie"

SERVES · 1
PREPARATION TIME · 5 MINUTES

1 tablespoon shredded or ribbon cut unsweetened coconut
3/4 cup coconut yogurt
2 teaspoons lemon juice
2–3 teaspoons raw honey, plus a drizzle to garnish
1/8 teaspoon pure vanilla extract
1 kiwifruit, peeled and sliced
1 heaping tablespoon gluten-free graham crackers (or regular naturally sweetened graham crackers), crushed
1 teaspoon finely grated lemon zest

Lemon and kiwifruit bring vitamin C and antioxidants to this bowl that emulates a cream pie. The yogurt tastes like custard and contains healthy fats, probiotics, and calcium. A toothsome crumble, made from gluten-free graham crackers, supplies a perfect finish for this "pie."

1 Place the coconut in a small saucepan set over medium heat and toast the coconut until it begins to brown. Remove from the heat and set aside.

2 Place the yogurt in a bowl and mix in the lemon juice, honey, and vanilla extract until combined.

3 Arrange or layer the kiwifruit and then the crushed graham crackers on top of the yogurt mixture. Garnish with the toasted coconut, lemon zest, and drizzle with a little honey.

PER SERVING	
Calories	407
Protein	3g
Fat	19g
Carbohydrate	67g
Sugar	36g
Dietary fiber	13g
Vitamins	C
Minerals	calcium

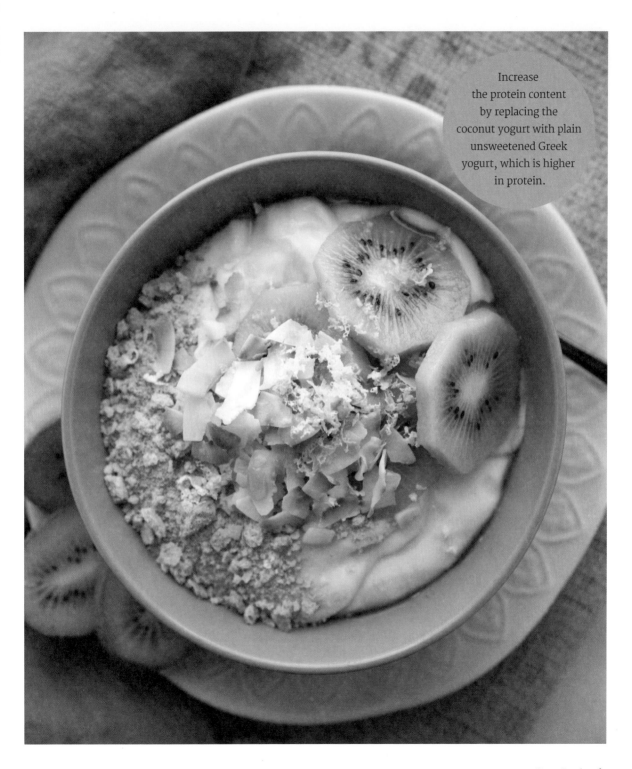

Increase the protein content by replacing the coconut yogurt with plain unsweetened Greek yogurt, which is higher in protein.

Try this!

Banana & Vanilla Cream "Pie"

If you love a traditional banana cream pie, then this bowl is for you. Banana is a great source of minerals, especially potassium, which plays an important role in muscular and digestive health, along with vitamin B_6, which supports a healthy nervous system.

SERVES · 1
PREPARATION TIME · 5 MINUTES

1 tablespoon shredded or ribbon cut unsweetened coconut
3/4 cup coconut yogurt
2–3 teaspoons raw honey, plus a drizzle to garnish
1/4 teaspoon pure vanilla extract
1/2 large, ripe banana, peeled and sliced
1 heaping teaspoon of hempseeds

1 Place the coconut in a small saucepan set over medium heat and toast the coconut until it begins to brown. Remove from the heat and set aside.

2 Place the yogurt in a bowl and mix in the honey and vanilla extract until combined.

3 Arrange or layer the banana and hempseeds on top of the yogurt mixture. Garnish with the toasted coconut and a drizzle of honey.

Try this!

Crispy Coconut & Caramel Cream "Pie"

If you've ever enjoyed the Girl Scouts' famous dark chocolate-drizzled, caramel and coconut-flavored cookies, you'll love this recipe. The combination of ingredients is divine, and they contain antioxidants and tons of flavor.

SERVES · 1
PREPARATION TIME · 5 MINUTES

1 tablespoon shredded or ribbon cut unsweetened coconut
3/4 cup coconut yogurt
2–3 teaspoons raw honey
1/8 teaspoon pure vanilla extract
1 tablespoon crushed pecans
1 tablespoon 70% dark chocolate shavings
1 heaping tablespoon crushed gluten-free graham crackers (or regular naturally sweetened graham crackers)

FOR THE CARAMEL SAUCE
1/4 teaspoon tapioca flour
2 tablespoons full-fat canned coconut milk
1 tablespoon pure maple syrup
1/4 teaspoon pure vanilla extract
pinch of sea salt

1 Place the coconut in a small saucepan set over medium heat and toast the coconut until it begins to brown. Remove from the heat and set aside.

2 To make the caramel sauce, combine the tapioca flour and coconut milk in a bowl and whisk until smooth. Heat a small saucepan over medium heat and add the coconut milk mixture, maple syrup, vanilla extract, and salt. Whisk continuously until smooth and bubbling. Simmer for 2–3 minutes, until reduced and slightly thickened, then remove from the heat and set aside.

3 Place the yogurt in a bowl and mix in the honey and vanilla extract until combined.

4 Arrange the crushed pecans, chocolate shavings, and crushed graham crackers on top of the yogurt mixture. Drizzle over the caramel sauce, then garnish with the toasted coconut.

Chocolate-Avocado Pudding

SERVES · 1
PREPARATION TIME · 35 MINUTES
COOKING TIME · 5 MINUTES

2 1/2 tablespoons 70% dairy-free dark
    chocolate chips or chunks
1 avocado, pitted and peeled
1 tablespoon cocoa powder
2 tablespoons unsweetened almond milk
1 tablespoon brown rice syrup
1/4 cup fresh berries

Avocado is an amazing source of essential fatty acids and is known to support skin and heart health, metabolism, and nervous system function. But you'd never know it was in this treat bowl! Here, avocado is blended with brown rice syrup, dark chocolate, and cocoa powder to create a creamy pudding.

1 Place 2 tablespoons dark chocolate chips in a heatproof bowl, set over a pan of simmering water, and stir until the chocolate is smooth and melted.

2 Transfer the melted chocolate to a single-serve blender or small food processor and add the avocado, cocoa powder, almond milk, and brown rice syrup. Blend or process until smooth.

3 Pour the mixture into a bowl and chill for 30 minutes.

4 When ready to serve, garnish the bowl with the berries and remaining 1/2 tablespoon of dark chocolate chunks or chips.

Try this!
Chocolate, Orange & Hazelnut

Chocolate and orange are a well-loved combination, thanks to the contrast of bright citrus and dark, rich, cocoa flavors. Here, hazelnuts add crunch and texture, too. Add 2 tablespoons of orange juice and 1 teaspoon of fresh orange zest to the ingredients in the blender. Garnish with segments of 1/2 an orange or tangerine and 2 tablespoons of chopped raw hazelnuts, instead of berries. Sprinkle with a pinch of sea salt to highlight.

PER SERVING	
Calories	380
Protein	5g
Fat	24g
Carbohydrate	44g
Sugar	22g
Dietary fiber	12g
Vitamins	C, B$_5$, B$_6$, E, K
Minerals	iron, magnesium

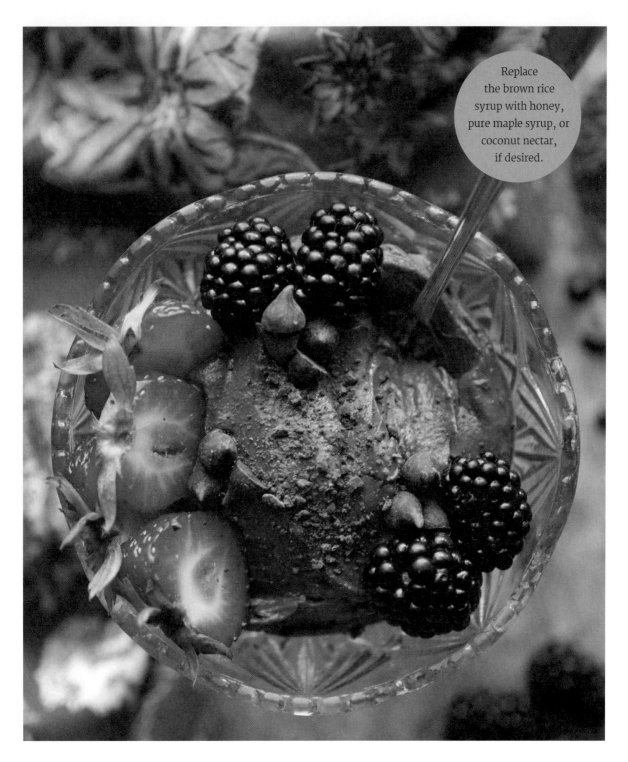

Replace the brown rice syrup with honey, pure maple syrup, or coconut nectar, if desired.

Warm Chia Berry Crumble & Coconut Cream

SERVES · 1
PREPARATION TIME · 3 MINUTES
COOKING TIME · 12 MINUTES

1/2 teaspoon tapioca flour
1 1/2 cups mixed frozen berries (blackberries, raspberries, strawberries, blueberries, etc.)
1 tablespoon chia seeds
1/2 tablespoon raw honey
1/4 cup naturally sweetened gluten-free granola
2 tablespoons coconut cream
a few fresh berries, to garnish

A warm bowl of fruit crumble topped with cream is a welcome treat on a chilly day. This bowl has all the qualities that make a fruit crumble delicious, but without the refined sugars and saturated fats. The fruits are sweetened with a little honey and granola, while pure coconut cream adds richness.

1 Place 2 tablespoons cold water in a small bowl and stir in the tapioca flour until it dissolves. Set aside.

2 Heat a large nonstick saucepan set over medium to high heat. Place the frozen berries in the warm pan, stirring slowly, until the berries begin to thaw. Cook for 3 minutes, then stir in the chia seeds, honey, and tapioca mixture.

3 Reduce the heat to medium and stir until the berry mixture begins to bubble and thicken. Reduce the heat to low and simmer for 5 minutes, until thickened. Transfer the berry mixture to a bowl.

4 Place the granola in a small saucepan set over medium heat and cook for 2 to 3 minutes, until it starts to get warm and crunchy. Remove from heat and place on top of the warm berry mixture. Drizzle with coconut cream and garnish with fresh berries.

PER SERVING	
Calories	361
Protein	7g
Fat	14g
Carbohydrate	56g
Sugar	29g
Dietary fiber	14g
Vitamins	A, C, K
Minerals	calcium, iron

Try this!
Warm Apricot Cinnamon Crumble

Swap out the berries for a different flavor combination—bananas and apricots. Omit the water and tapioca, chia seeds, and honey, and replace the berries with 1 sliced ripe banana and 2 sliced, small apricots. (Make sure the apricots are very soft and ripe.) Place the apricot, banana, and 1 teaspoon of olive oil in a saucepan with 1/2 teaspoon of cinnamon. Cook the fruit mixture for 3 to 4 minutes, until softened and combined into a thick fruit filling. Transfer to a bowl and complete the recipe as directed. You can garnish the bowl with chopped almonds or walnuts to add more crunch and healthy fats.

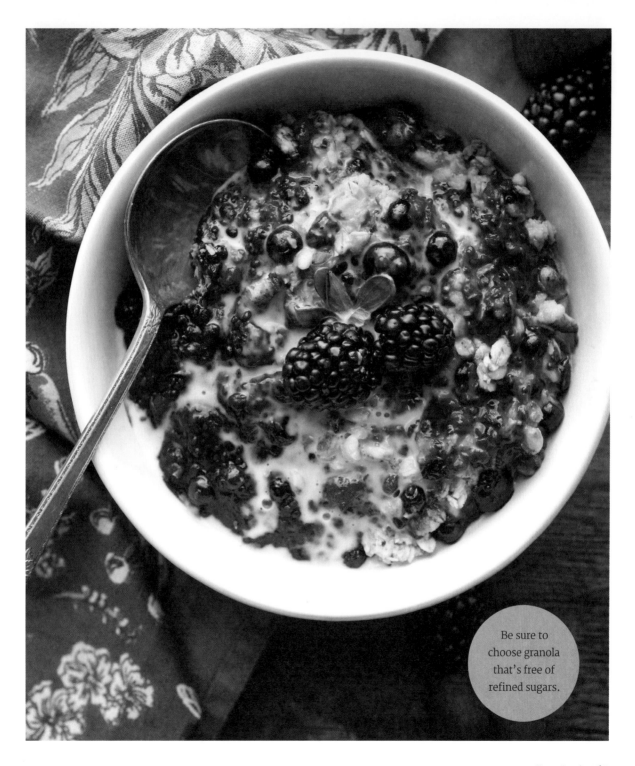

Be sure to choose granola that's free of refined sugars.

Vegan Blueberry Cheesecake

SERVES · 2
PREPARATION TIME · 7 MINUTES

1 (12-ounce) package organic non-GMO lite
  silken tofu
1 cup frozen blueberries
1 1/2 tablespoons pure maple syrup or
  coconut nectar
1/4 cup fresh blueberries
2 tablespoons crushed gluten-free graham
  crackers
2 teaspoons hempseeds
2 tablespoons raw walnuts
2 sprigs of fresh mint

Creamy, rich, and fruity, these cheesecake bowls are simple
to whip up and just as easy to eat! Silken tofu emulates
a rich cheesecake filling without the refined sugars and excess
calories, while supplying plenty of protein, calcium, and iron.
Plus, blueberries aid cardiovascular and cognitive health.

1 Combine the tofu, frozen blueberries, and maple syrup or coconut
nectar in a food processor and process until you have a smooth, pudding-
like consistency. Divide the mixture between two bowls.

2 Arrange or layer the fresh blueberries, crushed graham crackers,
hempseeds, and walnuts on top of the cheesecake mixture in each
bowl. Garnish with mint sprigs.

PER SERVING	
Calories	290
Protein	15g
Fat	10g
Carbohydrate	35g
Sugar	23g
Dietary fiber	3g
Vitamins	C, K
Minerals	calcium, iron

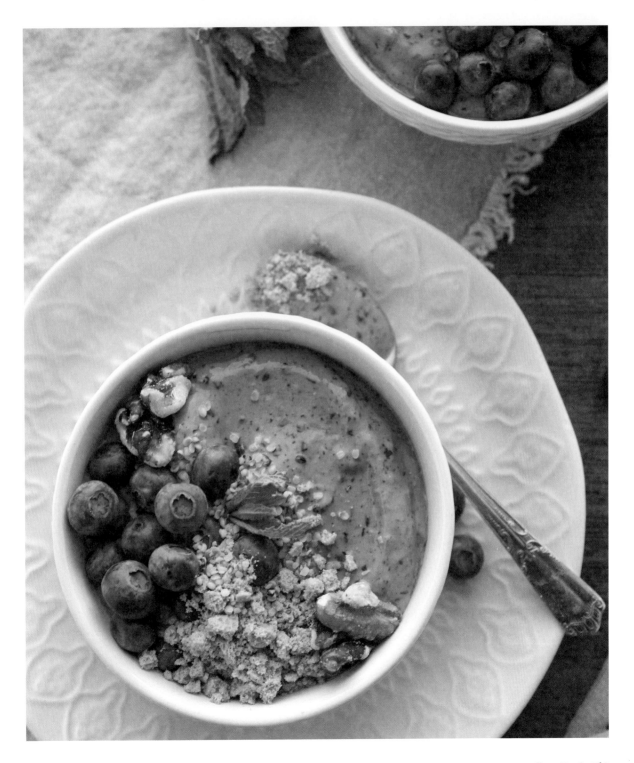

Try this!

Vegan Lemon Blueberry Cheesecake

Lemons are a true superfruit. Not only are they packed with vitamin C and antioxidants, they also stimulate the production of digestive enzymes—helping digestion for the whole day. This delicious fruit is also a powerful anti-inflammatory.

SERVES · 2
PREPARATION TIME · 7 MINUTES

1 (12-ounce) package organic non-GMO lite
   silken tofu
1¹/₂ tablespoons honey
¹/₄ teaspoon pure lemon extract
1 tablespoon fresh lemon juice
1 tablespoon finely grated lemon zest
¹/₄ cup fresh blueberries
2 tablespoons crushed gluten-free graham
   crackers
2 teaspoons hempseeds
2 tablespoons raw walnuts
2 sprigs of fresh mint

1 Combine the tofu, honey, lemon extract, lemon juice, and 1 teaspoon lemon zest in a food processor and process until you have a smooth, pudding-like consistency. Divide the mixture between two bowls.

2 Arrange or layer the fresh blueberries, crushed graham crackers, hempseeds, and walnuts on top of the cheesecake mixture in each bowl. Garnish with the remaining lemon zest and mint sprigs.

Try this!

Vegan Double Chocolate Cheesecake

This decadent double chocolate cheesecake is a must-try. Dark chocolate is indulgent, but it's also a superfood: It is rich in antioxidants and also contains magnesium and iron. Cocoa powder creates a rich, chocolaty flavor and enhances the dark chocolate.

SERVES · 2
PREPARATION TIME · 7 MINUTES
COOKING TIME · 3 MINUTES

FOR THE CRUST
3 soft Medjool dates, pitted
14 raw almonds
1/2 teaspoon cocoa powder
pinch of salt
1/2 teaspoon unsweetened almond milk

FOR THE CHEESECAKE
1 ounce 70% dairy-free dark chocolate
1 (12-ounce) package organic non-GMO lite
   silken tofu
1/2 tablespoon cocoa powder
1 1/2 tablespoons pure maple syrup or coconut
   nectar
2 teaspoons hempseeds
2 tablespoons raw walnuts
1 teaspoon of chopped or shaved 70% dairy-
   free dark chocolate

1 To make the crust, combine the dates, almonds, cocoa powder, salt, and almond milk in a small food processor and process until you have a crumbly, slightly sticky mixture. Scrape the mixture into a bowl and set aside.

2 Place the dark chocolate in a heatproof bowl and set it over a pan of simmering water. Stir until the chocolate is smooth and melted. Remove from the heat.

3 Transfer the melted chocolate to a small food processor with the tofu, maple syrup or coconut nectar, and cocoa powder. Process until you have a smooth, pudding-like consistency. Divide the mixture between two bowls.

4 Divide the chocolate crust between each bowl and garnish with the hempseeds, walnuts, and chopped or shaved dark chocolate.

Peanut Butter Cup Ice Cream

Ice cream is certainly a treat, but it is not the healthiest food. However, this dairy-free bowl contains a secret, healthy ingredient—frozen bananas. They make a delicious, allergen-friendly ice cream substitute. If you have a peanut allergy or intolerance, replace the peanut butter and nuts with almond.

SERVES · 2
PREPARATION TIME · 1 HOUR
FREEZING TIME · 1–2 HOURS

FOR THE PEANUT BUTTER ICE CREAM
3 medium bananas, frozen
1 heaping tablespoon natural peanut butter
1/4 cup full-fat coconut milk from a can
pinch of salt
2 tablespoons crushed roasted peanuts

FOR THE PEANUT BUTTER CUPS
1 tablespoon natural peanut butter
2 teaspoons coconut flour
1/2 teaspoon coconut palm sugar
2 tablespoons semisweet dark chocolate chips

FOR THE BOWLS
1 tablespoon crushed roasted peanuts
2 teaspoons hempseeds

1 To make the ice cream, combine the frozen bananas, peanut butter, coconut milk, and salt in a food processor. Process for 3 minutes, until you have a smooth, thick, and creamy mixture. Scrape the sides of the food processor with a spatula every 30 seconds or so. The mixture should resemble soft-serve ice cream.

2 Transfer the mixture to a loaf pan and fold in the crushed peanuts. Place the pan in the freezer for 1 to 2 hours, until firm. Check the ice cream from time to time, until it is the desired consistency.

3 Meanwhile, make the peanut butter cups. Combine the peanut butter, coconut flour, and coconut palm sugar and mix to combine. Place the bowl in the freezer for 10 minutes, until the mixture is firm.

4 Place the dark chocolate in a heatproof bowl and set it over a pan of simmering water. Stir until the chocolate is smooth and melted. Pour 1/4 to 1/2 teaspoon of the melted chocolate into the bottom of six candy-sized mini muffin liners.

5 Remove the peanut butter mixture from the freezer and divide it evenly between the muffin liners, placing it on top of the chocolate.

6 Pour the remaining melted chocolate evenly between the peanut butter cups. Then place the cups in the freezer to set.

7 When the ice cream and peanut butter cups are firm, remove them from the freezer. Divide the ice cream between two bowls. Remove the liners from the peanut butter cups and place three in each bowl. Garnish with the roasted peanuts and hempseeds.

PER SERVING	
Calories	442
Protein	9g
Fat	21g
Carbohydrate	59g
Sugar	31g
Dietary fiber	9g
Vitamins	B_6, C
Minerals	iron, manganese, potassium

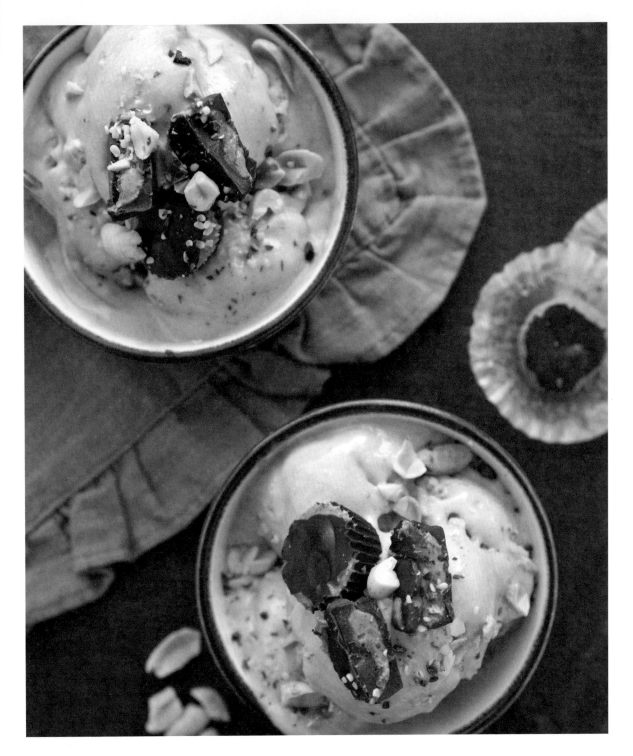

Try this!

Protein-Packed Nut Butter Cup Ice Cream

Increase the protein and swap out the peanut butter for another
nut butter, such as cashew or almond. Protein helps slow down
the release of sugars from carbohydrates in the blood-stream,
and also provides energy.

SERVES · 2
PREPARATION TIME · 1 HOUR
FREEZING TIME · 1–2 HOURS

FOR THE NUT BUTTER ICE CREAM
2 1/2 medium bananas, frozen
1/4 cup natural vanilla protein powder
1 heaping tablespoon natural cashew or
 almond butter
1/4 cup full-fat coconut milk from a can
pinch of salt
2 tablespoons crushed roasted cashews
 or almonds

FOR THE NUT BUTTER CUPS
1 tablespoon natural cashew or almond
 butter
2 teaspoons coconut flour
1/2 teaspoon coconut palm sugar
2 tablespoons semisweet dark chocolate
 chips

FOR THE BOWLS
1 tablespoon crushed roasted cashews or
 almonds
2 teaspoons hempseeds

1 To make the ice cream, combine the frozen bananas, protein
powder, nut butter, coconut milk, and salt in a food processor.
Process for 3 minutes, until you have a smooth, thick, and creamy
mixture. Stop every 30 seconds to scrape down the sides of the
food processor with a spatula.

2 Transfer the mixture to a loaf pan and fold in the crushed
cashews or almonds. Freeze for 1 to 2 hours, until firm.

3 Meanwhile, make the nut butter cups. Combine the nut butter,
coconut flour, and coconut palm sugar in a bowl and mix to
combine. Freeze for 10 minutes, until firm.

4 Place the dark chocolate in a heatproof bowl and set it over a pan
of simmering water. Stir until the chocolate is smooth and melted.
Pour 1/4 to 1/2 teaspoon of the melted chocolate into the bottom of
six candy-sized mini muffin liners.

5 Remove the nut butter mixture from the freezer and divide
it evenly between the muffin liners, placing it on top of the
chocolate layer. Pour the remaining melted chocolate evenly
between the nut butter cups, then place them in the freezer to set.

6 When the ice cream and nut butter cups are firm, remove
them from the freezer. Divide the ice cream between two bowls.
Remove the liners from the nut butter cups and place three
in each bowl. Garnish each bowl with the roasted cashews or
almonds and hempseeds.

Chocolate Strawberry Dream

SERVES · 1
PREPARATION TIME · 15 MINUTES
COOKING TIME · 5 MINUTES

1/2 ounce 70% dark chocolate, chopped
1/2 cup plain 0% fat Greek yogurt or coconut
  yogurt
1 teaspoon raw cocoa powder
1/2 tablespoon raw honey
1 tablespoon unsweetened shredded coconut,
  toasted
1/2 medium banana, sliced
1/2 cup strawberries, sliced
1 tablespoon chopped raw pecans

Chocolate and strawberries are a classic combination that creates a powerful antioxidant cocktail. Yogurt makes a rich and creamy base while honey adds natural sweetness that won't spike blood-sugar levels. Pecans add heart-healthy fats, minerals, and crunch. Depending on the yogurt used, this bowl can be dairy-free.

1 Place 1/4 ounce of the chocolate in a heatproof bowl and set it over a pan of simmering water until melted. Transfer to a serving bowl and stir in the yogurt, cocoa powder, and honey. Chill for 10 to 15 minutes.

2 When you are ready to serve, remove the mixture from the fridge and arrange the toasted coconut, banana, strawberries, and pecans on top of the bowl. Garnish with the remaining 1/4 ounce chopped chocolate.

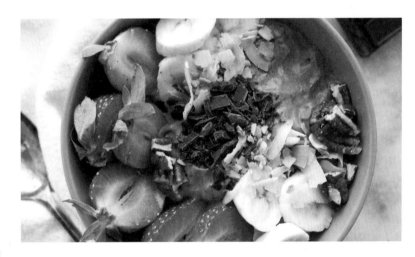

PER SERVING	
Calories	355
Protein	15g
Fat	16g
Carbohydrate	45g
Sugar	27g
Dietary fiber	8g
Vitamins	C
Minerals	calcium, iron, potassium

Try this!
Almond Pistachio Frozen Yogurt

Create a frozen yogurt with a different flavor profile. Omit the cocoa powder and plain chocolate. Blend the yogurt and honey with 1/4 teaspoon pure almond extract, 1/2 medium frozen banana, 1/4 cup raw spinach, the flesh of 1/4 avocado, and 3 ice cubes until smooth. Then freeze for 2 to 3 hours, until the consistency of frozen yogurt. Serve garnished with 1/3 cup sliced banana and 2 tablespoons raw pistachios.

Lemon Poppyseed Trifle

SERVES · 1
PREPARATION TIME · 15 MINUTES

FOR THE CURD
½ cup plain 0% fat Greek or coconut yogurt
½ tablespoon raw honey
1 tablespoon fresh lemon juice
1 tablespoon lemon zest
⅛ teaspoon pure lemon extract
⅛ teaspoon pure vanilla extract

FOR THE CRUMBLE
3 tablespoons raw cashews
5 soft dates, pitted (about 1 ounce)
1 tablespoon almond flour
1 tablespoon coconut flour
1 tablespoon lemon zest
1 tablespoon fresh lemon juice
⅛ teaspoon pure lemon extract
⅛ teaspoon pure almond extract
⅛ teaspoon pure vanilla extract
1 teaspoon poppyseeds
½ tablespoon unsweetened almond milk

FOR THE BOWL
2 or 3 fresh raspberries
twist of lemon zest

PER SERVING	
Calories	403
Protein	19g
Fat	15g
Carbohydrate	50g
Sugar	34g
Dietary fiber	7g
Vitamins	C
Minerals	calcium, iron, magnesium

These layers of a creamy lemon "curd," separated by a fiber-rich, protein-packed crumble, are the perfect light, citrusy dessert. The curd is a yogurt mixture sweetened with honey, while the crumble combines nuts, dates, poppyseeds, coconut flour, and lemon. Depending on the yogurt used, this bowl can be dairy-free.

1 To make the curd, combine the yogurt, honey, lemon juice and zest, and lemon and vanilla extracts. Mix well until smooth. Place in the fridge to chill, while preparing the crumble.

2 Combine all the crumble ingredients in a food processor. Process on low for 30 seconds to 1 minute, until the mixture forms sticky crumbs.

3 Remove the lemon curd mixture from the fridge. Place one-third of the crumble in the bottom of a separate bowl, then place half the curd on top. Place another third of the crumble on top of the curd and top with the remaining lemon curd. Finish with the remaining crumble. Garnish with raspberries and a twist of lemon zest.

Try this!
Peanut Butter Brownie Trifle

A rich, chewy chocolate brownie crumble, layered with creamy peanut butter yogurt, makes a surprisingly healthy treat. Peanuts are full of minerals, including iron and magnesium, plus they supply protein and healthy fats. They pair well with the dark chocolate, which adds antioxidants and richness. For the curd, replace the lemon juice, zest, and extract, and vanilla extract with ½ tablespoon natural peanut butter and chill in the fridge while you make the crumble. To make the brownie crumble, replace the cashews with raw almonds, and the coconut flour, lemon zest, juice, and extract, almond and vanilla extracts and poppyseeds with 1 tablespoon almond flour, ½ tablespoon cocoa powder, and 1 tablespoon 70% dark chocolate chips. Layer the crumble and curd, as directed, and garnish with raspberries.

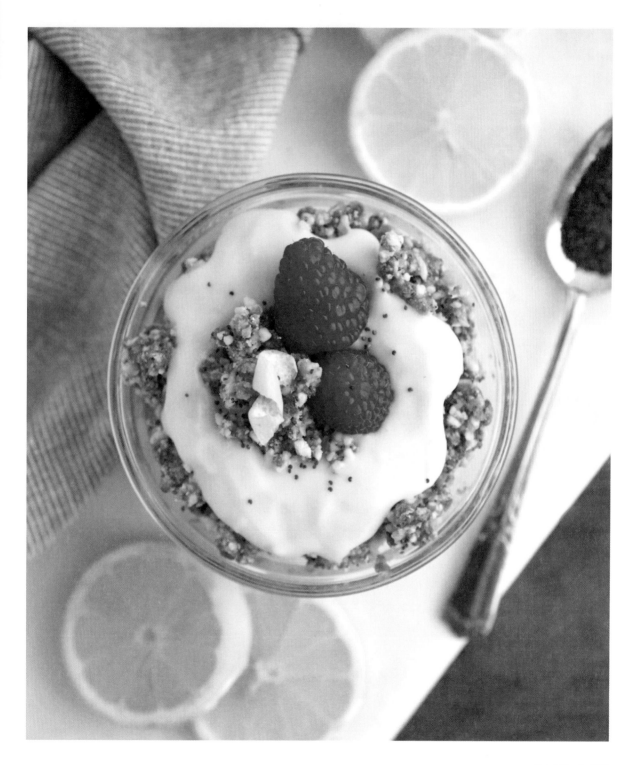

Black Forest Cake Chia Seed Pudding

SERVES · 1
PREPARATION TIME ·
4 HOURS 10 MINUTES

FOR THE CHERRY CHIA SEED PUDDING
2 1/2 tablespoons chia seeds
1/2 cup unsweetened almond milk
1/2 tablespoon raw honey
1/2 cup frozen cherries

FOR THE CHOCOLATE PUDDING
1/4 ounce 70% dark chocolate
2 tablespoons vanilla Greek or coconut
   yogurt
1/2 teaspoon cocoa powder

FOR THE BOWL
1 tablespoon coconut cream
1/4 ounce 70% dark chocolate, shaved
2 fresh raspberries
2 fresh cherries

This pudding replicates all the delicious components of a Black Forest cake in a healthier, fiber-loaded treat. The key ingredients are the chia seeds, which are particularly beneficial to the digestive system.

1 To make the cherry chia seed pudding, combine the chia seeds, almond milk, and honey in a bowl and mix well. Cover and chill in the fridge for 4 hours, or overnight, until thickened.

2 Combine the thickened chia pudding and cherries in a blender or food processor and blend for 1 to 2 minutes. Transfer the mixture to a serving bowl.

3 Place the chocolate in a heatproof bowl and set it over a pan of simmering water. Stir until the chocolate is smooth and melted. Transfer the melted chocolate to a small bowl and stir in the yogurt and cocoa powder, until smooth. Spoon on top of the cherry chia pudding.

4 Place the coconut cream on top of the chocolate mixture and swirl it into the cherry chia and chocolate pudding mixtures with a spoon. Garnish with the shaved dark chocolate, raspberries, and cherries.

PER SERVING	
Calories	344
Protein	8g
Fat	19g
Carbohydrate	342
Sugar	22g
Dietary fiber	15g
Vitamins	-
Minerals	calcium, iron, magnesium

Try this!
Caramel Apple Pie Chia Bowl

Take the flavors of a classic apple pie—soft apples, aromatic cinnamon, sugar, and a flaky, buttery crust—add caramel and chia seeds, and you have a guilt-free treat to enjoy. Replace the cherries with 1/4 cup unsweetened applesauce and 1/4 cup diced fresh apple; reduce the almond milk to 1/4 cup and add 1/4 cup natural apple juice and 1 teaspoon ground cinnamon. Mix all of the ingredients together and let them thicken in the fridge for 4 hours. Omit the chocolate pudding. Stir the chilled and thickened apple pudding and transfer it to a serving bowl, top it with 2 tablespoons vanilla Greek or coconut yogurt and 2 tablespoons of granola, a pinch of ground cinnamon, and finish with a drizzle of caramel sauce (see Crispy Coconut & Caramel Cream "Pie," page 163).

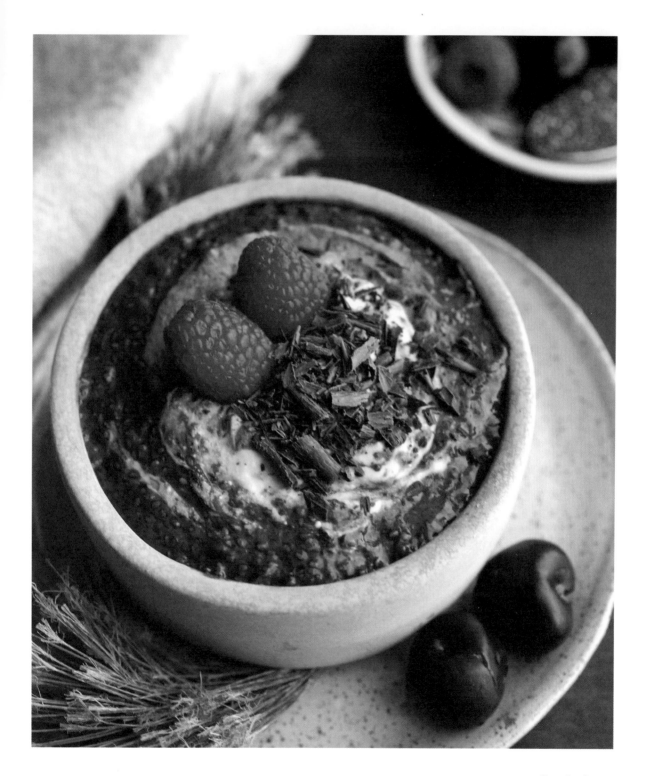

Creamy Carrot Cake

SERVES · 1
PREPARATION TIME · 10 MINUTES

FOR THE MAPLE CREAM CHEESE SWIRL
1/2 tablespoon regular cream cheese or
   dairy-free cream cheese, softened at room
   temperature
1/2 tablespoon pure maple syrup
1/2 tablespoon unsweetened almond milk

FOR THE CARROT CAKE BASE
1/4 cup diced raw carrot
1/2 cup frozen pineapple
1/2 cup frozen peaches
2 tablespoons coconut cream
3/4 cup unsweetened almond milk
2 soft dates, pitted
1/2 teaspoon ground cinnamon
1/4 teaspoon ground nutmeg
1/4 teaspoon ground ginger

FOR THE TOPPINGS
1 teaspoon pistachios, crushed
1 teaspoon hempseeds
1 teaspoon chopped walnuts
1/2 tablespoon raisins
pinch of cinnamon

Carrot cake's rich cream cheese frosting, combined with the dense cake, is a terrific marriage of savory and sweet. This bowl contains all of the flavors of the dessert, along with vitamins, fiber, and antioxidants. Depending on the cheese used, it can be dairy-free.

1 To make the maple cream cheese swirl, place the cream cheese in a bowl and aerate it with a wooden spoon. Stir in the maple syrup. Add the almond milk, a little at a time, stirring continuously, to make a smooth mixture. Set aside.

2 To make the carrot cake base, combine the carrot, pineapple, peaches, coconut cream, almond milk, dates, cinnamon, nutmeg, and ginger in a high-speed blender. Blend until thick and smooth.

3 Transfer the cake mixture to a bowl. Drizzle the bowl with the cream cheese mixture and cut through it with a knife to create a feather pattern.

4 Garnish with the crushed pistachios, hempseeds, walnuts, raisins, and cinnamon.

PER SERVING	
Calories	359
Protein	6g
Fat	16g
Carbohydrate	52g
Sugar	41g
Dietary fiber	8g
Vitamins	A, C
Minerals	calcium, iron

Try this!
Protein-Packed Creamy Carrot Cake

Bring a little more protein power to this tasty treat by adding protein powder to the carrot cake base. The powder will make the bowl even more satisfying, give your body a boost of amino acids, help keep blood-sugar levels stable, and may even help stimulate your metabolism. Replace the coconut cream and dates in the carrot cake base with 1/4 cup of your favorite natural grass-fed whey or plant-based vanilla protein powder (with no artificial sweeteners, flavors, or additives) and increase the almond milk to 1 cup. Complete the recipe as directed.

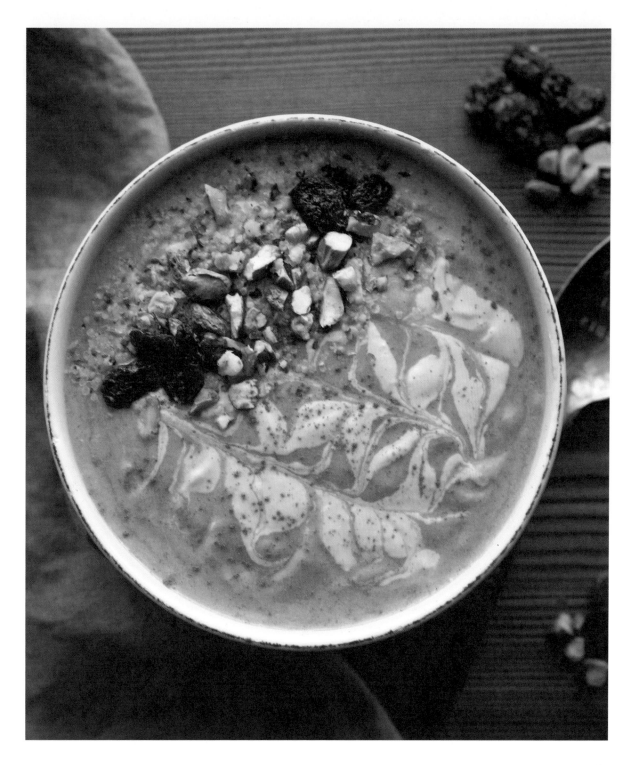

Power Bowl Extras

Use the information in this chapter when you want to substitute an ingredient in one of the recipes, find a local or online supplier, or convert ounces to grams.

Ingredient Substitutions

If you have an allergy or intolerance to an ingredient used in a power bowl recipe—or just don't enjoy eating it—here are some alternatives you can use.

Dairy Substitutes

1 oz Cheddar or feta cheese = 1 oz dairy-free cheese

1 tablespoon cream cheese = 1 tablespoon dairy-free cream cheese

1 tablespoon sour cream = 1 tablespoon plain Greek yogurt or 1 tablespoon dairy-free sour cream

1 tablespoon mayonnaise = 1 tablespoon Vegenaise

1 cup almond milk = 1 cup cashew milk, rice milk, coconut milk (carton, not canned), hemp milk, soy milk, cashew milk, hazelnut milk, 1% cow's milk (if tolerated)

1 cup plain Greek yogurt = 1 cup plain coconut yogurt, plain soy yogurt, plain almond yogurt, plain cashew yogurt

Grain Substitutes

1/4 cup buckwheat groats = 1/4 cup chopped nuts of choice or 1/4 cup of your favorite granola

3 1/4 oz dry buckwheat (soba) noodles = 3 1/4 oz dry brown rice noodles, black bean noodles, mung bean noodles

1/2 cup uncooked rolled oats = 1/2 cup uncooked quinoa flakes

1 cup cooked whole-grain pasta = 1 cup cooked rice pasta, corn pasta, quinoa pasta, gluten-free blend pasta or 3/4 cup cooked rice, 3/4 cup cooked quinoa

Egg Substitutes

1 whole egg = 1/4 cup crumbled extrafirm organic tofu (in dishes where eggs are scrambled)

Other Ingredient Substitutes

1 teaspoon chia seeds = 1 teaspoon ground flaxseeds

1 teaspoon hempseeds = 1 teaspoon chia seeds, whole flaxseeds

1 cup cooked quinoa = 1 cup cooked rice, millet, or amaranth

1 cup arugula = 1 cup watercress

1/2 cup black beans = 1/2 cup kidney beans, chickpeas, edamame beans, navy beans

1 cup chopped or torn kale = 1 cup chopped Swiss chard

1 cup cooked sweet potatoes = 1 cup cooked potatoes of choice

1/2 cup blueberries = 1/2 cup raspberries, diced strawberries, blackberries

1 tablespoon coconut palm sugar = 1 tablespoon granulated cane sugar, turbinado sugar

1 teaspoon honey = 1 teaspoon agave nectar, coconut nectar, pure maple syrup

1/2 cup cooked chicken breast = 1/2 cup cooked turkey breast or 1/2 cup shelled edamame beans

1 breakfast sausage link = 1/4 cup cooked ground chicken or turkey breast

1 tablespoon almond butter = 1 tablespoon natural peanut butter, cashew butter, sunflower butter

1 tablespoon almond flour = 1 tablespoon hazelnut flour

Conversion Charts

Oven Temperature

°F	°C
225	110
250	120/130
275	140
300	150
325	160/170
350	180
375	190
400	200
425	220
450	230
475	240

Weights

STANDARD	METRIC
1/2 oz	15g
1 oz	27g
11/2 oz	40g
2 oz	55g
3 oz	80g
31/2 oz	95g
4 oz	110g
5 oz	140g
6 oz	175g
7 oz	200g
8 oz	225g
9 oz	255g
10 oz	285g
11 oz	310g
12 oz	340g
13 oz	370g
14 oz	400g
15 oz	425g
1 lb	450g
11/4 lb	550g
11/2 lb	680g
2 lb	900g
21/4 lb	1kg
21/2 lb	1.1kg

Measures

STANDARD	METRIC
1/4 in.	5mm
1/2 in.	1cm
3/4 in.	2cm
1 in.	2.5cm
11/4 in.	3cm
11/2 in.	4cm
2 in.	5cm
3 in.	7.5cm
4 in.	10cm
6 in.	15cm
7 in.	18cm
8 in.	20cm
9 in.	23cm
10 in.	25cm
11 in.	28cm
12 in.	30cm

Liquids

STANDARD	METRIC
1 tsp	5ml
1 tbsp	15ml
1/8 cup	30ml
1/4 cup	60ml
1/3 cup	80ml
1/2 cup	120ml
2/3 cup	160ml
3/4 cup	180ml
1 cup	240ml
2 cups	480ml

Resources

Many of the ingredients used in *Power Bowls* can be found in some supermarkets, including organic proteins and fresh produce, whole grains, nuts, and seeds. However, if you have difficulty tracking any of them down, you should be able to find them in specialty stores or online suppliers.

USA

NATURAL AND ORGANIC FOODS STORES

Fresh Thyme Farmers Market
freshthyme.com

Sprouts Farmers Market
www.sprouts.com

Trader Joe's
www.traderjoes.com

Whole Foods
www.wholefoodsmarket.com

REGULAR STORES WITH NATURAL AND ORGANIC FOODS SECTIONS

Albertson's
www.albertsons.com

Food Lion
www.foodlion.com

Hannaford
www.hannaford.com

Harris Teeter
www.harristeeter.com

Publix
www.publix.com

Safeway
www.safeway.com

Target
www.target.com

Wegmans
www.wegmans.com

ONLINE GROCERY SUPPLIERS

Amazon
www.amazon.com

iHerb
www.iherb.com

Manitoba Harvest
https://manitobaharvest.com

Mountain Rose Herbs
www.mountainroseherbs.com

Navitas Naturals
www.navitasorganics.com

Sambazon
www.sambazon.com

Canada

NATURAL AND ORGANIC FOODS

Planet Organic (Edmonton, Calgary)
planetorganic.ca

Whole Foods
(Vancouver, Ontario)
www.wholefoodsmarket.com

Blush Lane Market (Edmonton)
www.blushlane.com

BULK NUTS/SEEDS/DRIED FRUITS

Bulk Barn (throughout Canada)
www.bulkbarn.ca

REGULAR STORES WITH NATURAL AND ORGANIC FOODS SECTIONS

Real Canadian Superstore (throughout Canada)
www.realcanadiansuperstore.ca

Save-On-Foods (British Columbia and Alberta)
www.saveonfoods.com

Sobeys (throughout Canada)
www.sobeys.com

Safeway (throughout Canada)
www.safeway.com

ONLINE

Amazon
www.amazon.ca

Spud
www.spud.ca (Vancouver, Calgary, Edmonton)

Vitamart
www.vitamart.ca

UK

NATURAL AND ORGANIC FOODS

Grape Tree
www.grapetree.co.uk

Holland & Barrett
www.hollandandbarrett.com

Planet Organic
www.planetorganic.com

Whole Foods
www.wholefoodsmarket.com

ONLINE

Amazon
www.amazon.co.uk

Australia

NATURAL AND ORGANIC FOODS

Fundies Wholefood Market
www.fundies.com.au

BULK NUTS/SEEDS/DRIED FRUITS

The Source Bulk Foods
thesourcebulkfoods.com.au

ONLINE

Amazon
www.amazon.com.au

Aussie Health Products
www.aussiehealthproducts.com.au

Honest to Goodness
www.goodness.com.au

New Zealand

NATURAL AND ORGANIC FOODS

Piko Wholefoods
www.pikowholefoods.co.nz

ONLINE

Naturally Organic
www.naturallyorganic.co.nz

Index

Picture Credits

All images taken by Christal Sczebel, copyright Toucan Books Ltd., except:

p.56 Getty Images/DigitalVision Vectors, bubaone; p.80 Getty Images/DigitalVision Vectors, fonikum; p106 Getty Images/iStock, Panptys; p.132 Getty Images/iStock, Panptys; p.156 Getty Images/DigitalVision Vectors, appleuzr; p.182 Getty Images/DigitalVision Vectors, appleuzr. Additional icons, p.7, courtesy of Leah Germann.

Author Biography

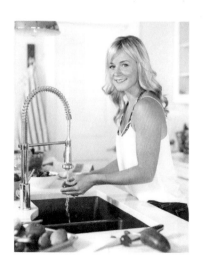

Christal Sczebel is a Certified Holistic Nutritional Consultant, based in Edmonton, Alberta, Canada. She is the owner of a private nutrition practice called Pure & Simple Nutrition with a team of practitioners focused on helping their clients discover optimal health through nutrition and sustainable wellness. Christal is also the owner and author of Nutrition in the Kitch (www.nutritioninthekitch.com), a website filled to the brim with her recipe creations, food photography, and a selection of online nutrition guides and programs that help readers reach their best health through nutrition and living well. She published her first cookbook in 2017.

Acknowledgments

Creating my second cookbook has been an incredibly fun journey and so many people have helped me along the way. First and foremost, I have to thank God, who has blessed me with amazing opportunities, given me strength to push through, and gifted me with an incredible love for health, food, writing, and photography.

To my hubby Justin for his constant support and willingness to taste-test every recipe I create (even the ones that end up in the "fail pile").

To my family and friends, my faithful fan club that always encourages me, offers to help, and—of course—also volunteers for taste-testing.

To my fellow nutritionists and bloggers, who inspire me to stay ambitious and keep working at what I love.

And to the editors, designers, and other professionals, who made the pages of this book come together seamlessly.

Thank you!